So Far,
So Good

*A Memoir of a Brain Tumor
Patient and His Caregiver*

Kathy Beechem

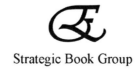

Strategic Book Group

Strategic Book Group
P.O. Box 333
Durham CT 06422
www.StrategicBookClub.com

ISBN: 978-1-60976-995-6

Typography and page composition by J. K. Eckert & Company, Inc.

This book is dedicated to my husband,

Peter Thomas Nadherny.

The bravest person I know.

Contents

Acknowledgments

Thank you to the early readers of my manuscript. You provided me much needed encouragement and helpful feedback. Mike and Mary Jo Whelan, Betty Rushing, Todd Olson, Barb Seibel, Dr. Ron Warnick, Stephanie Beechem, Ricki Collins, and Bill Dillon. Each of you provided a unique perspective of the journey recorded here.

Thanks to my niece, Shauna Whelan, who early on helped me find my "voice" and showed me I was writing a memoir.

Thanks to Dianne Powers who cleaned up the pictures in this book so they could be acceptable to the publisher. A tedious task performed with love for Pete and me!

Thanks to Christine Duque who helped me with my technological challenges with word processing and readied the manuscript for submission. Your time and attention to detail is so appreciated.

1

What Was

"So Far, So Good" was how my husband, Pete Nadherny, would answer the question, when asked by someone, "How are you doing?" They would not be asking casually. Pete had discovered he had a brain tumor on December 20, 2005. "So far, so good" was a new phrase for him. He had not used it before. This phrase reflected how Pete dealt with his diagnosis, surgery, subsequent recovery and treatments. "Today, I am OK," he was saying to those who asked. "I have come this far on my journey. I am not sure how many more days I will have, but I have today, and it is good."

Pete owned a successful small business, which did executive search work for local and national companies. It was called "The Angus Group" and was located in Cincinnati, Ohio, our home since the early Eighties. Pete and his partner, Dave Hartig, had bought out the previous owner and had been running it successfully for the last twelve years. The company did about a million in revenue, and had a staff of ten other professional recruiters. Pete was the Chief Executive Officer and focused his attention on business and staff development.

Pete was the super coach of his team, and was proudest of the people he had developed who worked with him. Pete generated the most billings in the firm. He had been honored for a number of years by his peer group, winning many Pinnacle awards which was a national recognition for top billings in a given category or industry. Dave focused on the administrative functions of the business, and generated the second-highest billings. They complemented each other well and liked working together.

Pete had been a human resources professional his whole career, having worked in large corporations in Chicago, Illinois; Jacksonville, Florida; Washington, DC and Cincinnati, Ohio, before he decided to open his own business fifteen years ago. His father, who died when Pete was eleven years old, had also been a human resources professional for a large company in Chicago. Pete was an only child. His mom and dad had him late in life. A nice surprise. They had given up the possibility of ever having children by the time they were in their late thirties. Pete was born premature at a total weight of three-and-one-half pounds. His mother and father loved him madly. As only mature parents with a single child can do, they showered him with nice clothes and travel to places throughout the world. His love of travel and nicely tailored clothes came from them.

Pete lost his Mom three years after his dad died. Both parents had died at the age of fifty-one years. Pete was only fourteen years of age. Pete was greatly influenced by his loss of them. He fought anxiety about being abandoned most of his adult years. He vowed to have children when he was young, so they would never have to experience abandonment like he had. And he did. By age twenty-five, Pete had two wonderful sons, Michael and Steven. By the time Pete discovered his brain tumor, they were adults in their thirties; Michael was living in Florida and Steven was living in Washington, DC.

I was in my late twenties when I met Pete. At first, it was his professional success and competence that attracted me. I loved working with him. I came to trust his judgment and perspective on business issues. I was an overly confident and highly critical young professional at the time, and not many business people had earned my respect. I loved his high standard of performance both for himself and others. He challenged me regularly, and immediately began investing in me to develop me and coach me to become better at what I did. His ethics and honesty were without question. He was driven to be his best, and committed to making our company the best.

Pete loved boats and we owned a thirty-five-foot cruiser, which we kept on the Ohio River. The Ohio River runs through downtown Cincinnati. Most of our social activities from May through October each year were centered on the boat. Our home, in a city neighborhood, Mount Adams, overlooked the river. Pete loved the water. He knew all the barges that traversed the river. He had taken hundreds of pictures of them over the years, always with a watchful eye for the unique and different. I framed pictures of the Ohio River barges one year for his birthday.

Pete also had a passion for sports cars. He had owned over a dozen Porsches throughout the years, always buying used ones, since the price of a new one was exorbitant. He took great pride in his selection of the "right" used Porsche. In his late twenties and early thirties, Porsches were Pete's hobby. He participated in a number of concourses with his used Porsches. A concourse is a competitive event where car owners show their cars, much like dog owners show their dogs. Concourse winners show a compulsion for car cleanliness, authenticity of parts, paint, and devotion to detail not easily imagined by the average person.

Pete had given up participating in concourses by his early thirties, because being that compulsive was not really in his nature. However, Pete still enjoyed participating in Porsche Club events. He was over his concourse phase by the time he and I were married, but we competed quite well in numerous Porsche-sponsored car rallies over our twenty years of marriage. The trophies in our dining room attest to the events where Pete won with me as his navigator. I came to love Porsche rallies. What better way to spend a beautiful Saturday or Sunday afternoon than riding around with the top down in our Porsche, driving fast on the country roads in Ohio? In the year 2000, we made a trip to Stuttgart, Germany, to buy our first new Porsche. A new Porsche was a dream comes true for Pete. We picked our car up at the Porsche factory, and got it up to one hundred and forty miles an hour on the autobahn later that same day. It was a thrill of a lifetime for both of us. I still drive that car.

As Pete's wife, I worked as an executive of a bank. It was a national bank, and I had responsibilities for the bank's retail business in over twenty states. I had eleven thousand people working in my group. I traveled at least three days a week every week. I had a hectic, demanding schedule. I had gained a lot of recognition in the banking industry, having been named as one of the "Twenty-Five Most Powerful Women in Banking" in the United States by a trade magazine the year before Pete discovered his tumor.

Pete was truly not just my partner in life, but also in my career. He was my advisor and coach. On a personal level, Pete did all those tasks that I didn't take the time to do: getting both cars serviced, letting in the window cleaners, managing any home construction projects, paying the bills and taking out the garbage. I couldn't have had the success I had at the bank if it hadn't been for Pete's support. I bragged about him to my staff and colleagues. He supported me, and never made me feel guilty for the sixty-five plus hours I would work each week. He attended every bank event when invited, so Pete was well known to my staff and other executives in the bank.

When we were at home we did everything together. We went to the grocery store together, ran Pete's errands to his favorite spots like Home Depot or Sears, and went to the wine store. Socially, we were always together. Rarely would either of us go out without the other for a social occasion. We had never vacationed without the other.

Pete loved going to fine restaurants for dinner, and he enjoyed his wine. Wine was his hobby, and he was knowledgeable about American wines and growing regions. I did business in San Francisco, so between bank events in Napa and my business trips to San Francisco, we made half-dozen visits to Napa over the last five years. Pete would readily join me for a quick weekend. He never tired of the wineries. Based on his research in wine trade magazines, we always had a list of "must visit" wineries for our next trip. He kept detailed notes. I could tell you today every winery we ever visited.

Pete and I had a great marriage based on a genuine partnership. We loved each other deeply, and never tired of each other's company. I guess other people would have called us soul mates, even though we had never used this term to describe ourselves. When Pete was diagnosed, we had been married twenty years.

Neither Pete nor I were born into a life of privilege. Born in Chicago, Pete was made a guardian of his Mom's sister Aunt Belle and Uncle Ed, after his Mom and Dad died. Pete's parents' life insurance had provided Pete a college education, which was not automatic in his family by any stretch. His aunt and cousins were so proud of the high degree of professional success Pete had achieved. They respected his intelligence, hard work, and leadership of others. Pete loved his Aunt Belle, and took on the many duties of an only son after his Uncle Ed died. Belle died at age eighty-five in 1997. Prior to her death, Belle suffered from a form of Alzheimer's. Pete and I made monthly trips to Chicago for many years to take Belle to the hair salon and the grocery store, clean the house, manicure the lawn and do any home improvements necessary. Pete was faithful. We never skipped a trip, regardless of the weather. I still remember the day Belle died. I was doing business in Columbus, Ohio, and Pete called me on my cell phone to tell me. I sped home and found him packing his suitcase, weeping like a child whose heart had been broken.

When Pete was diagnosed with his brain tumor, his family was made up of his one surviving aunt, Violet, in Chicago, several cousins in the Chicago and the Detroit areas, his sons, Michael and Steven, Steven's wife Kathy, and me.

I had grown up in the Cincinnati area. My mother and father had six children, and had raised us on my dad's civil servant salary. My mother never worked outside of our home. They sacrificed a lot to send us to Catholic elementary and high schools, believing sincerely in the power and safety of their faith, and entrusting their children to Catholic school teaching. We had lots of love in our home growing up, but not a lot of extras. My siblings and I still laugh about our addiction to bacon and orange juice. They were highly desirable by us as children, but rationed carefully. Each of my siblings and their families lived in the Cincinnati area, except for my brother, Joe, and his family, who lived in Eugene, Oregon.

Our family gatherings meant thirty-plus people showing their affection for each other rather loudly, with lots of hugs. Pete, although at first overwhelmed with this clan, had begun referring to all those "Beechems" as his family too, the longer we were together. Pete had been adopted by my family, and was loved as a brother and son.

I had been raised Catholic, but left any affiliation with the institutional church over twenty-five years ago. I had always seen myself as a spiritual person, and had dabbled in New Age readings. I was a lone ranger and liked it that way. I was introspective and had a contemplative side to my nature. I had kept a personal journal for most of my life, and God was always an important part of my thinking. Over the last several years, as my relationship with God had grown, my journal became a prayer journal, and I used it daily.

Pete was not an overtly religious person. He had been raised Catholic, and had attended Sunday school. His former wife had been a Christian Scientist, and he had always rejected that religion. Neither he nor his sons had any regular religious practices or traditions.

Early in the year 1999, as I was praying one morning, I was struck by my own arrogance. In my journal, I wrote, "What am I thinking? How do I think that I can have an independent relationship with God without any advice or support from others?" Ouch! I recognized the truth. I felt shame. I believed this insight was indeed from God. "OK," I wrote. "I'll find a church community. If I want to grow closer to God, I need to find a community to grow in."

I told Pete after boating season was over that year that I was going to search out a church. I told him exactly what happened and why.

Did he want to come with me? I asked. He said, "Yes." I was so surprised and delighted. That simple yes was one of the best gifts he ever gave me. To share the search with him was so different than me searching alone. It now became part of our adventure together. And so Pete and I went church shopping in the fall, and after visiting six or seven churches found a community called Crossroads that was Christian, contemporary and non-denominational. It was a church for the un-churched, and perfect for us. We have both been engaged with that community ever since.

Pete rarely talked about his relationship with God, but he loved our new community as much, if not more, than I did. It had great contemporary music. The teaching pastor was slightly irreverent, and a man's-type man. Pete loved him. Now, with this news about his tumor six years later, Pete expressed a deep faith. From that first night when we talked about the full body scan results, and the possibility that he had a brain tumor, Pete would respond to my worries or anxiety by simply and repeatedly saying, "We'll see what the Lord wants." And that was it. I sensed a peace from him. He expressed little anxiety.

2

This Changes Everything

Pete knew lots of people in the business community in Cincinnati, where we lived and worked. It was his business to know people. He probably interviewed over five hundred people a year. In early fall of 2005, I had chartered a boat out of Newport, Rhode Island, to take Pete, me, Michael, Steven and their significant others on a cruise around Cape Cod and the islands. Pete and I were boaters. Pete's two sons had grown up on boats. It was my way of celebrating Pete's six-tieth birthday in a way that would most please him. It was an expensive vacation, more than we had ever paid before. On that trip, Pete had trouble remembering the name of Michael's girlfriend. He was so afraid of offending her! Both sons noticed, and began to tease him. Shortly after we got home, Pete made an appointment with his primary care doctor. He was also having trouble remembering names of his candidates, and would come home from work with a three-by-five index card in his shirt pocket with the names of the candidates and clients he had seen that day. His primary care doctor referred him to a psychologist. Both doctors told him he was just growing old. "Memory loss just happens when you turn sixty," they said.

That was in late fall. But Pete knew something wasn't right. He didn't talk much about it, but he must have mentioned it enough that I had noted his worry over forgetting names in a letter to a good friend of mine that October of 2005. I discounted most of his concern, though. Pete was a very cautious man, and I thought he was just being his overly cautious self. He had compensated for any name lapses so well, I did not notice any change in our life. Neither had his colleagues at the Angus Group.

"A sign is a change that is evident to another person. A symptom is something that you as a patient feel and describe as being abnormal," writes Peter Black in *Living with a Brain Tumor.* There were no signs with Pete. None of us who knew him suspected anything seriously wrong. But Pete knew something was wrong.

Other brain tumor victims have had more severe symptoms than the occasional name lapses Pete experienced. Others have suffered severe headaches, sometimes with nausea or vomiting. Others have had seizures, which can be a more dramatic call to action. However, like Pete, others may experience minor changes, like a slight weakness or numbness in one side of their body, or occasional vision blurriness or difficulty with concentration. Many times, the symptoms are not specific to a brain tumor.

With Pete, I quickly learned to trust his assessment of his own body. He knew. And throughout our journey, when so many others, including medical staff and sometimes members of the family, wanted me to take charge of the decision-making for Pete, I resisted. I trusted Pete's knowledge of his own body and what he needed.

Pete discovered his own brain tumor. He scheduled his own full-body scan MRI in late December of 2005. No doctor's order. No insurance. He paid for it himself. Charged it to our credit card. Cost him fifteen hundred dollars. He had casually mentioned to me that he was going to get the scan done. I was in an all-day meeting the day he went. By the time I came home that evening, he had already called my sister Mary Jo, the resident nurse in our family, with the results. Can you imagine the radiologist's reaction when a spot showed up in Pete's brain that was about one and a half inches long, and very bright on the MRI? The radiologists told him to wait after the scan was complete. Pete sat in the waiting room all alone. "I knew then that something was wrong," he told me later that evening.

"Something is showing up in your brain on the scan. It looks bad. The rest of your body is fine," the technicians told him. "It could be a brain tumor," they told him.

Pete said he felt numb. He went silent. They told him he needed to see a doctor right away. They recommended the Mayfield Group. Pete went back to the office.

I came home about 7:30 that night, and he was sitting in his normal place in our living room reading the newspaper. I remembered that he had had the scan that day, and casually asked what he learned. He turned his face to me. Tears welled up in his eyes.

"They found something," he said. "They think it is a brain tumor. It is in the left temporal lobe."

It was December 20, 2005. I can remember the scene like it was yesterday. I went over to his chair, got down on my knees, put my arms around him and laid my head on his chest. We held each other in a long embrace. Tears streamed down both of our faces. Finally, I said: "This changes everything." And it had.

"This changes everything" was actually a decision that I made in a split second. There were probably a million ways I could have responded to Pete's news. I look back on that decision now, and think God's hand was all over it. I wasn't fearful at that moment, or full of pity for me or Pete. I just recognized in that instant that everything that had been our life had just changed. We suddenly needed to re-evaluate everything in our life according to new criteria. I didn't know what those new criteria were at the time, I just knew it wasn't what was. In an instant, I felt a detachment from things that twenty-four hours before had seemed so important and worthy of my atten-tion. The tasks of my job at the bank. My volunteer commitments. All those faded in color. What burnt bright for me was researching infor-mation about brain tumors and treatment.

For Pete, the house suddenly became pre-eminently important. He started making lists of the things that needed to be done, and he tack-led the list with urgency. For both of us, we couldn't get enough time together. We started planning how to spend more time with friends. Pete made a list of old friends he hadn't seen for awhile. We couldn't spend enough time at Crossroads.

As I started researching information on brain tumors and their treatment, I felt wave after wave of fear. I had difficulty catching my breath. I had a pounding in my stomach, the muscles tightening and releasing every time I read things like "brain tumor patients have a two percent survival rate." I found myself deep breathing a lot to release the tension such information created in me.

Pete had no interest in researching any information. At first, I'd share everything I was learning, but slowed that process down as I saw his complete lack of interest. Pete showed deep sadness and dis-appointment. He was easily touched by others' kindness to him. He cried easily. A man whom I had seen cry only two or three times in the last twenty-five years now was easily moved to tears. Welled-up-in-the-eye tears. Leaky tears. Not sobbing tears. Pete would say, "My eyes are misty."

Pete had called my sister, Mary Jo and her husband, Mike, before I had gotten home the day he got his news, and shared the information with them. They were the only ones who knew. By the time we called them back that same night, Mary Jo had already started her research. She was feverishly at work. Pete was touched by her responsiveness to his circumstance, and the work she and Mike in a few short hours had already done on his behalf. His eyes filled with tears as he listened to what they had learned.

Pete was adamant about not wanting anyone else to know about the possibility that he had a brain tumor. He didn't want to ruin Christmas for others. Pete's graciousness; the consummate gentleman! I couldn't believe it, but I respected his wishes. Neither of us told anyone else: neither our sons and other family members, nor colleagues at either of our companies. Mary Jo, Mike, Pete and I huddled on the phone that night and for days afterwards. It reminded me of the war council calls the bank would have when considering an acquisition, when we all shared information about what we had discovered in our fact-finding due diligence.

Our first task was to find a doctor. The radiologists where Pete had gotten his scan done had suggested the Mayfield Group in Cincinnati. Mike was on the website naming the doctors listed when Pete said, "Oh, I know the president of the Mayfield Group. I did some work for him a few years ago. I'll call him and get his best referral."

All of us on the phone smiled. Pete at his best! Pete called Mike Gilligan, the president of the Mayfield Group. Mike told Pete that, in his opinion, Ron Warnick was the best surgeon in town. Pete scheduled an appointment with Dr. Warnick for December 28, 2005. We checked out Dr. Warnick ourselves. Mary Jo was a registered nurse, knew medical people, and knew how to access resource information only available to medical personnel. She quickly discovered that Dr. Warnick had a very good reputation. One evening during one of our phone huddles, Mary Jo reported her research on primary brain tumors.

- Primary tumor means the tumor originated in the brain, not metastasized from a cancer somewhere else in the body.
- About 100,000 people a year get the unexpected diagnosis of a brain tumor; approximately 40,000 of those are like Pete's, origi-

nating in the brain. The rest have spread from cancers in the lung, colon, breast, or elsewhere.

- White males over fifty are the most common target for primary brain tumors.
- Gliomas are the most common type.
- There are four grades of glioma tumors based on the aggressiveness of their growth.
- The left temporal lobe, where Pete's tumor was located, is one of the four major parts of the brain, and regulates memory, emotions, hearing, language and learning.

We scoured through information on the websites of the American Cancer Society, Brain Tumor Society, National Brain Tumor Foundation, American Brain Tumor Association, and Clinical Trials and Treatments for Brain Tumors. I ordered books. Pete was strangely detached from our flurry of activity, other than joining in on the phone calls when we reported our findings. It was almost as if he was the bystander. I became the researcher and information gatherer, along with my sister. Pete had almost no interest in what we were learning, although when developing the list of questions before that first doctor visit, Pete added a few of his own.

Our immediate set of questions included:

- How is a real diagnosis made?
- Do you ask for a biopsy first before surgery?
- Surgery seemed the most common and first treatment. Do you do a biopsy before or as part of the surgery?
- Radiation and chemotherapy seemed part of the "standard treatment." What are the side effects of all that?
- Gamma knife surgery was done on some brain tumors. That is a much less invasive procedure. Is that something Pete could consider?

The two most helpful books I found were by Dr Paul Zeltzer: *Brain Tumors: Finding the Ark,* and its companion *Brain Tumors: Leaving the Garden of Eden.* These books were written with the patient in mind, and chock-full of good information.

I was so eager in my information gathering, because I was searching for some hopeful answers. There were none. Maybe Pete already knew that. His detachment from our information search might have reflected how difficult it was for him to embrace the facts of this disease. His mind and his spirit just couldn't deal with any more information.

There was no known cause for brain tumors. There were lots of hypotheses about possible causes from things like cell phone use, weakened immune system, and bad genes, but no definitive answer. Brain tumor patients and their families didn't need to spend any time feeling guilty about things they could have done to prevent the tumor. There was no known cause. There was also no known cure. All that could be done was treatment options.

In those early days I felt like I was being punched in the gut each time I read words like cancer, malignant, craniotomy, two percent survival rate. What an awful disease! A few people did survive for more than five years, which is the researchers' way of defining a cancer survivor. But the percentages were working against the brain tumor patient. Both Pete and I saw quickly that the prognosis was bad, and that a real battle was in front of us. Although terrified, I never lost hope. There are always a few survivors. Why couldn't Pete be one of them!

I looked at, and started talking about, dealing with Pete's brain tumor as a new adventure for us. It seemed like an appropriate word. Pete and I had been on adventures previously in our lives. When we used that word previously, it implied a little risk, but lots of opportunity. When Pete decided to go into business for himself, it was an adventure for us. When we bought a house and moved into the city from the suburbs, it was an adventure. Joining Crossroads was an adventure. Now it was Pete's health that was at risk, and that risk had launched both of our lives into a new world with strange language and different terrain. It was unfamiliar. A high sense of urgency filled the air in our house.

An adventure is defined by the American Heritage dictionary as "an undertaking of a hazardous nature; participation in a course of events marked by excitement and suspense." Yes, we had hazard and suspense. We had embarked on a journey not of our own choosing, that had a high probability of a bad outcome. Was there also great opportunity? I felt like I was preparing for the fight of our lives. In the midst of this danger, Pete felt peace. So did I. We weren't panicked. Both of us went back to work the following days and weeks. We had always felt safe as long as we were together. We knew we were in this adventure together.

From my prayer journal: December of 2005

> Lord, what do you want of us in this journey? How we need you.
> Give us your loving grace and presence. Help me to be a source of

comfort, advice, and support to Pete. I need you so! I won't do well without you. I'll be a jerk. Too self-centered. I'll miss your clues and Pete's clues. I'll not hear. I'll be unresponsive.

I lift Pete to you. We trust you. Sanctify Pete. Sanctify me in this circumstance. Make me a worthy servant of Pete & you. Let me know more of you through serving him.

3
Diagnosis

Pete and I had made it through Christmas with lots of joy, and our secret still a secret. We hosted my big family of over thirty people Christmas night at our house for dinner. We had set up a special treat that night: a taped interview with my Mom and Dad, seventy-nine and eighty-four years old, respectively. The children, grandchildren and great-grandchildren piled into our home with their questions ready.

"Where were you born? What grade school did you go to? Tell us about how you snuck into Wrigley Field to watch Roger Hornsby play. What did your Mom and Dad do for a living? What part of Chicago did you live in?" The conversation went on for a couple of hours.

What a magnificent time we had. Pete and I stayed up to the early morning hours, cleaning and recovering from that party. I would look at him repeatedly through the holidays working so hard, and full of so much life and energy. How could he have a brain tumor? For a few hours, both of us forgot about the heavy burden we carried.

But now it was December 28, the date Pete had scheduled to see Dr. Warnick at the Mayfield Clinic in Cincinnati. It was only eight days since Pete had his initial scan done, but it felt to me as if years had passed. So much had changed.

Mary Jo went with us. Dr. Warnick was the chairman of the American Association of Neurological Surgeons' Section on Tumors

(AANS). He had received the National Brain Tumor Foundation Award for Excellence in Research, and the Mahaley Clinical Research Award from the AANS. Dr. Ron Warnick walked into the treatment room, and Pete immediately recognized him, as did Ron recognize Pete. It was like a surprise meeting of old friends at an event. Pete smiled a huge smile.

"We met at Leadership Cincinnati," Pete and Ron said almost in unison. I saw Pete relax. A friend!

Dr. Warnick put the scans of Pete's MRI on a lighted screen in the treatment room. We saw the culprit: a four-centimeter blob of white light in the left temporal lobe of Pete's brain. The doctor said it looked like a tumor that was about one-and-a-quarter inch deep. It was a primary tumor, meaning that it originated in the brain. The doctor said he guessed it was about three to six months old, and was growing very fast. He said he was about ninety percent certain it was a glioblastoma multiforme, and that it was malignant. There appeared a darkened area in the center that looked like necrosis (dead tissue), which was characteristic of glioblastomas.

Dr. Warnick said, "There was nothing to gain by observing. A biopsy would tell us what it is for sure, but a biopsy would not remove the tumor. The best treatment was to remove the tumor. The surgery could be done safely."

He estimated he could get between eighty to ninety percent of the tumor out. He would then follow the surgery with radiation once a day for six weeks, joined with Temodar, an oral chemotherapy.

We knew that this was the standard treatment protocol for treatment for GBMs (glioblastoma multiforme tumors) after surgery, from the research we had done. The doctor wanted a more detailed picture, what he called a functional MRI, which would help him determine the degree of risk, and what language areas could be affected during surgery. He promised to take Pete's scan to the Tumor Board that upcoming Wednesday. Experts from all over the city would review Pete's MRI, and Pete would get the benefit of their opinion.

> "Most hospitals have at least one tumor board. This is a group of doctors, nurses, administrators, psychologists, and other interested professionals who gather regularly for an hour or so to discuss recent cases. Their meetings begin with a formal written history that details how the diagnosis was made, pertinent examinations, surgical results, laboratory findings, and scan reports. Test results are usually presented by experts in specific areas. The neuroradiologist will present findings from MRI scans; the neurosurgeon will discuss surgical out-

comes, observations and diagnostic impressions. It is a great advantage for patients to have their case presented at a tumor board meeting. At what other time could all treating physicians be together to focus or discuss a case with all the pertinent information available? It's like getting ten to fifteen consults at no charge."

−Brain Tumors: Leaving the Garden of Eden

Throughout Pete's illness, Pete had the benefit of having his case reviewed by the Brain Tumor Boards at both the Cleveland Clinic and in Cincinnati on a monthly basis.

Dr. Warnick immediately put Pete on the anti-seizure medication Keppra, and a medium dose (eight mg) of decadron, a steroid, to prevent swelling in Pete's brain. He told Pete drinking could trigger a seizure—so he had to have a dry New Year's Eve. Dr. Warnick wanted to schedule Pete's surgery for the week of January 9 or 16. We asked about risks of the surgery.

"It is rare that anyone dies during brain surgery," Dr. Warnick said. "The risks were to your verbal dictionary, comprehension, and/ or vision that could be affected due to the location of the tumor. It's possible, Pete, that after surgery, you might never be able to drive again."

On that first doctor visit Pete weighed one hundred and sixty-seven pounds. Pete responded calmly. He was his friendly self as he shook Ron's hand, thanked him, and left the office.

Dr. Warnick seemed so matter-of-fact to me with Pete. He was very professional. He just said it looks like this, therefore the procedure is this, blah blah. I wanted to scream. I wanted him to tell us "This looks really bad! Yeah, Pete, this could kill you! You could die from this tumor, and you could die fast." Why hadn't he said that? I wondered. The only way I could tell the graveness of the situation was by how quickly Dr. Warnick wanted the follow-up MRI, and how quickly he wanted to schedule surgery. Nothing in the medical world had ever moved this fast before, in my experience.

I had approached that doctor visit with fear and dread. The dread was appropriate. It was about as bad as it could get. The doctor was fairly sure that Pete had a Grade IV Glioblastoma Multiforme (GBM) tumor. The only worse thing would have been if the tumor had been in a position that made it inoperable. "GBM is a rapidly progressing cancer that invades brain tissue and can impact physical activities and mental abilities. It affects about 6700 persons in the United States every year. Following initial treatment with surgery, radiation and/or chemotherapy, the cancer nearly always returns" (FDA News, May 8, 2009). Pete looked to be one of those sixty-seven hundred.

My fear led me to lift Pete to God in prayer. I asked for Pete's full restoration right then. "Make him whole," I prayed. I frequently began to have a very intense picture of God in my imagination as the source of life: abundant, green, rich life, like a rain forest in the midst of the desert. I imagined this God of abundant life healing and restoring Pete completely—not marginally, but completely. I'd tell God that I knew he didn't do things half-way; when he healed, he did it fast and completely.

Diagnosis of a brain tumor is a difficult thing. It can only really be determined after the tissue is taken out of the brain where the tumor is through surgery, and then studied by a pathologist who can determine if the tissue is cancerous. Pete and I never really questioned Dr. Warnick's diagnosis. It looked like a tumor to him on the MRI, and it could be operated on, given its position in Pete's brain. We understood why the doctor wanted it removed as soon as possible, because it would continue to grow fast and damage good brain tissue, as well as create swelling and pressure in all parts of Pete's brain. So the biopsy that determined that the tumor was cancerous, and what type of cancer it was, would be done after Pete's tumor was already removed.

An MRI (magnetic resonance imaging) gave Dr. Warnick the best picture of a brain tumor as compared to an X-Ray or a CT (computed tomography) scan. An MRI was used for lots of medical conditions, but for a brain tumor it was the most relied-upon tool. Pete had over thirty MRIs in a two-year period. These pictures became the primary way the doctors monitored what was happening in Pete's brain with the tumor. The MRI provided detailed images of the brain in three dimensions, at many different angles and different levels. The resulting picture, which could be projected on a computer screen, showed great contrast between different soft tissues in the brain. By adding a dye called gadolinium, which is usually administered during the MRI intravenously, the cancerous tissue looked extremely bright. Normal tissue didn't light up. Pete and I always said "white is not a good color" on an MRI.

An MRI was not a painful procedure. Pete would remove his belt, watch and glasses, since any metal on the body or in the body (staples, metal pins, etc.) was not allowed in the MRI scanner. It was usually very cold in the room so Pete layered up, and the technicians were ready with blankets. Pete would go feet-first into the scanner.

The scanner covered his whole body. It was a dark and enclosed space. The technicians would talk to Pete during the scan to get a better picture when his brain was active. "They won't even let me sleep," Pete complained in a teasing sort of way. There would be a loud clanging sound throughout the test. It usually took between forty-five minutes to an hour. The technicians came to love Pete, and he loved them back. They were very kind to him. He never complained about his MRIs.

From my prayer journal: December 28, 2005

The doctor is today, Lord. I guess it is natural to expect the worst. I put my trust in you. I lift Pete into your hands. Fill me with your spirit to be your loving presence and comfort to him. I praise you for all the wonderful things you have done for us and given us. Your presence, your spirit, makes every day, every event, super-charged with life. Give us your empowerment, that we may live this day with full hearts. You gave your son so we may have life—life forever with you. I accept your gift! How lucky we are. No other God but you. You restore all life. You renew. Give Pete your grace and restore him.

4

Second Opinion

I contacted my brother, Dr. Joe Beechem, a PHD biophysicist who was doing cancer research, about Pete's diagnosis and proposed surgery. I asked him to check his sources and share what he knew about brain cancer treatment. Immediately he began finding sources for alternate treatments for Pete. He raised the prospect of gamma knife surgery, which wouldn't be so invasive. He had a good contact at the University of Pittsburgh. Joe encouraged us to get a second opinion.

Pete messaged Dr. Warnick about getting a second opinion. Dr. Warnick said that the gamma knife procedure was probably not appropriate for Pete's tumor at this initial stage, but if we wanted a second opinion, he would encourage us to get one. He gave us doctor names at the Cleveland Clinic; M.D. Anderson in Houston, Texas; U.C. San Francisco; and a colleague at the Mayfield Clinic. All were national brain tumor centers, except the Mayfield Clinic. Cleveland was just a drive away. The decision was easy for Pete and me. We were off.

We decided to fly to Cleveland for the second opinion on January 11, 2006. This was less than two weeks since Pete's initial diagnosis on December 28 from Dr. Warnick. I was surprised at how easy it was to get an appointment. Everything had changed now. Whenever we told doctors of Pete's situation, or when anyone looked at his MRI or test results, we got action. Appointments. Call-backs. Prescriptions.

We experienced this level of responsiveness throughout Pete's journey. Pete and I laughed about how this was a good thing and a bad thing. We never experienced frustration from waiting on a doctor call back, which was a good thing; the bad thing was the extreme seriousness of Pete's condition that triggered this responsiveness.

We were to see Dr. Eugene Barnett, the director of the Brain Tumor and Neuro-Oncology Center at the Cleveland Clinic. He and Dr. Warnick were friends. We stayed at a hotel right on the campus of the Cleveland Clinic. The clinic was one of the highest-rated hospitals in the country. It is one of the national centers for research and treatment of brain tumors. The Brain Tumor Institute participated in numerous national clinical trials. If some treatment was being tested for treatment of brain tumors, they either were participating or knew about it. All the staff at the Brain Tumor Institute specialized in brain tumor treatment, whether they were nurses, oncologists, researchers, pathologists or radiologists.

The Cleveland Clinic campus was a campus. It went on for blocks. Dr. Barnett was in a newly constructed Neurology Center that was beautiful and big. The reception desk was like a main library, and was a little intimidating with its presence and professionalism. The staff was very friendly and helpful. Dr. Barnett's nurse clinician, Gail, had been with Dr. Barnett a long time. She did a full medical history and a neurological exam of Pete. The neurological exam results were normal. Pete weighed 159 pounds by the time we got to the clinic. He had lost ten pounds since the visit with Dr. Warnick.

Dr. Barnett confirmed Dr. Warnick's assessment. He was matter-of-fact, but kind. He spent over an hour with us. He spoke very calmly. Pete's mass was deep in the left temporal lobe, about one-and-a-half inches long. It was near the hippocampus, but not in a difficult area to get to from a surgical perspective. He thought that it looked like a glioblastoma multiforme (GBM) tumor due to the dark area in the center, which was dead tissue and was characteristic of glios. He explained our options: observe, drugs, radiation or surgery/biopsy. Experimental treatments were not really available until it was determined what the tumor was for certain.

He thought he could get about ninety-five percent of the tumor out through surgery. He talked about whether to do the surgery awake or asleep. He said Pete wouldn't need to have all of his hair clipped, just two to three inches where the incision would be made. He would use a micro-surgical technique, taking off the anterior tip of the temporal lobe. Pete would probably be released from the hospital two to four days after surgery. In seven to ten days the pathology results would be back, and we would have a definite diagnosis. Standard care was then six weeks of radiation with a low dose of Temodar, which was an oral chemotherapy.

Dr. Barnett rattled off the risks of the surgery in response to our questions. There was a high chance of losing some of Pete's peripheral vision in the upper right quadrant. Forty to fifty percent of the patients with tumors located where Pete's was lost their ability to drive. Dr. Barnett thought some of Pete's memory was probably gone from the damage the tumor had already done, given where it was. Speech could be affected, too, by surgery. About fifteen to twenty percent of the patients' speech was worse off after the surgery. About five percent of brain tumor patients have understanding affected, as well as speech. Five percent of them experience some paralysis on the right side. About one percent of the time, the surgery results in a vegetative state. Heart attacks, viruses, pneumonia and blood clotting tend to go with having a brain tumor. Gamma knife surgery has shown no effectiveness with a GBM.

Dr. Barnett talked of three clinical trials going on at the clinic which Pete might be eligible for. The big problem with brain tumors was that you can get the tumor out through surgery, but there are cancerous cells in and around the tumor bed that can't be seen, and can't be surgically removed. So brain tumors recur most of the time.

Dr. Barnett spoke most enthusiastically about one of the trials that used an immunotoxin called IL 13-pe38qqr. He explained that the cells of a glioblastoma multiforme tumor have lots of IL-13 receptors, which normal brain cells don't have. This IL-13 immunotoxin latches onto these cells with the receptors, killing the cancer cells, but not the normal brain cells. The toxin would be inserted into Pete's brain through catheters in a second surgery, which had to happen fourteen days after his tumor was removed. The toxin had to drip into Pete's brain through these catheters for ninety-six hours. Then, after this second surgery, a standard care treatment of radiation and Temodar would be prescribed. He described this as a two-step process. Pete could have the actual brain tumor removal surgery done by Dr. Warnick in Cincinnati, and then come to the clinic for the IL-13 trial. We asked Dr. Barnett for his assessment of Dr. Warnick's skill as a brain surgeon. He leaned back in his chair and smiled.

"If my mother had a brain tumor and she lived anywhere close to Cincinnati, Dr. Warnick would be my choice to operate on her," Dr. Barnett said.

Pete and I laughed. Enough said.

Pete was sitting across from me during the visit with Dr. Barnett. He looked like he was in a business meeting. His legs were crossed and his portfolio was opened, and he was taking notes. Pete asked the hard question toward the end of the conversation: "What are my chances?"

Dr Barnett answered, "If your tumor is a GBM, and since you are over sixty, the outcome is not very good with conventional treatment. Fifty percent of the patients live eleven months; the other fifty percent live less than eleven months, normally three to six months. Fifteen percent of GBM patients live two years. The clinical trials are somewhat more promising. These treatments can affect some people very positively, and extend their life." Dr. Barnett replied matter-of-factly, but with kindness.

Pete's body jumped, like he had just received an electrical shock from a bad outlet, as Dr. Barnett rattled off these statistics. I was sitting across the room. My heart was breaking. Pete just kept taking notes.

I felt like I was having a nightmare that just wouldn't end. Bad news and more bad news. Pete's face reflected the nightmare: shock; pain; sadness.

"I thought I might have more like a couple of years. Not months!" he said to me as we left.

I felt so tense. How do I prepare for this? How does Pete prepare? How do I help him get ready for death?

We learned through our journey that brain tumors were as unique as the people who had them. No two are alike. If you had a brain tumor, statistics didn't really speak to your individual situation. The same treatment would affect two patients in very differing ways with varying results. The location of your tumor, your age, your genetic makeup, your overall health, and past medical history all influenced the effectiveness of any given treatment.

We felt so glad to have gotten a second opinion. The experience that the Cleveland Clinic team of doctors and staff have had with different types of brain tumor patients gave us confidence that they would probably have had experience with someone with symptoms or effects Pete might likely have. It was a huge relief to think of them being on our side. Being a national center, they were able to administer many different types of treatments, versus a less experienced team that may be wed to the treatment for which they were either funded or had researched.

Pete's first question to Dr Barnett was: "How many brain surgeries do you do a year?"

"Over a hundred," he said.

Our rule was not to have anyone do brain surgery on Pete unless they did at least a hundred brain surgeries a year. From our research, we knew the skill of the neurosurgeon matters. As *Brain Tumors: Finding the Ark* explains: "A neurosurgeon's skill can be defined as a 'numbers game.' There are about 30,000 primary brain tumors diagnosed yearly in the United States and there are about 4,500 active neurosurgeons. This means that all things being equal, the average neurosurgeon would operate on six to seven patients a year. But we know that each of the nation's twenty largest centers operate on more than two hundred primary brain tumors annually. Thus, the majority of surgeons see far fewer than six to seven cases a year. Survival times and quality of life for people undergoing neurosurgery in high volume centers were dramatically better in centers having fifty or more surgeries per year."

Pete's one hundred brain tumor surgeries requirement was probably too conservative. Any surgeon who had done fifty surgeries a year would have assured us an experienced hand. Dr. Barnett had passed our test. So had Dr. Warnick.

There were many brain tumor centers that did second opinions for free, and many second opinions that I could access through the institution's website. I had sought, in addition to the Cleveland Clinic, second opinions from both U.C. San Francisco and Duke University later in Pete's treatment cycle.

> "Your plans after the second opinion can be affected in at least three ways:
>
> 1. Your current assessment and treatment plans are confirmed.
>
> 2. You get new treatments or courses of action which your current doctors can implement for you. Or
>
> 3. You may have more confidence in the new team and switch for this stage in your care."
>
> *–Brain Tumors: Leaving the Garden of Eden*

We felt a little uncomfortable seeking a second opinion, because we feared that our first doctor, Dr. Warnick, would be offended, and interpret our search as a lack of confidence in him. Stories of doctors with big egos, who are easily angered, filled our imagination. But only our imagination. Those fears were unfounded in our experience. We know that this is not true for many patients. We have heard stories of doctors refusing to see patients if they had obtained a second opinion, or refused to treat them unless the patient made an either/or decision. We were spared this suffering. We couldn't have had a more cooperative relationship between the two doctors if we had designed it ourselves. Both Pete and I interpreted this cooperation as a God-thing—one of his early miracles with Pete. Here's what happened.

Two days after our visit to the Cleveland Clinic, Pete, Mary Jo, and I visited Dr. Warnick. It was January 13, 2006. We went to this visit having decided to have Pete's surgery completed in Cincinnati by Dr. Warnick, and then travel to the Cleveland Clinic for the clinical trial treatment of the IL-13. The clinical trial would increase Pete's life expectancy from a three percent chance of living more than eleven months to a twenty-five or thirty percent chance. Pete and I did not have a hard time making these types of decisions. Both of us had run businesses, and were used to making decisions fast and frequently, with the best information we could gather in the time we had. We expected to set a surgery date with Dr. Warnick at this visit, and get the results from the Cincinnati Tumor Board Review held earlier in the week.

We got surprised. Drs. Warnick and Barnett had already talked extensively about Pete by the time we went to see Dr. Warnick. Dr. Warnick recommended that we go to Cleveland and have everything done by Dr. Barnett.

"Dr. Barnett will be better equipped to do the catheter placement for the IL-13 treatment if he removes the tumor himself," Dr. Warnick explained. "Your chances of getting into the clinical trial are greater if Dr. Barnett does the surgery. There are only two places left in the study. If Dr Barnett doesn't do the surgery, you may find that there is no place left for you by the time you want the procedure done. To increase your chances to live longer, I'd recommend you have the surgery done and the IL-13 treatment done by Dr Barnett."

Pete protested. "Couldn't we have you do the surgery here, and wait until you have approval for the clinical trial you will conduct here with the Gliadel wafers?"

"I believe in any brain tumor treatment that uses a convexion therapy, which is what IL-13 does," Dr. Warnick said. "Same principle of treatment as the gliadel wafers, Pete. You can increase your chances to live for more than eleven months from three percent to twenty-five or thirty percent by participating in this trial." Dr. Warnick paused and looked compassionately at Pete. Then he softly said, "Pete, you don't have the time to wait for Mayfield to get approved for our clinical trial. You need to act now."

Pete moved right to the decision. "Of course, let's do it. The Cleveland Clinic it is," he said.

I was struck by how unselfish Dr. Warnick was. How motivated he was for Pete's best interest. And I was struck by the cooperation of these two doctors—Ron Warnick at the Mayfield Group in Cincinnati really talking with Gene Barnett from the Cleveland Clinic about Pete Nadherny, and what was the best course of action to take for him. I knew enough about the medical system to know that this kind of cooperation from senior people from well-established institutes was very unusual.

"I think we just witnessed our first miracle," I told Pete.

This cooperation between Cincinnati and the Cleveland Clinic continued throughout all of Pete's treatment, sometimes with new and different players—making it all the more miraculous.

Pete's friend Bill was waiting in the parking lot for Pete as we walked out. Bill took Pete to lunch. Bill had arranged for Pete to have an alternative treatment experience called Healing Touch with a highly skilled healer who was an associate of Bill's. Bill was a Healing Touch practitioner, but was young in terms of his experience. He wanted Pete to have the best!

I went back to work. I didn't know at that time that Friday, January 13 would be the last day I would ever work for the bank. I spent that afternoon talking to the project manager for the clinical trial using IL-13 at the Cleveland Clinic. Her name was Deb, and she scared me thoroughly. She kept telling me to think about it.

"There are a lot of risks," Deb kept saying. "Pete might not even qualify; depends on how he does in the first surgery. We will test him after the first surgery to see if he qualifies. This trial is tightly controlled because it is a national study. No, you can't get the radiation done in Cincinnati; you'll need to have everything done at the clinic."

The conversation went on and on. I got her to fax the papers I needed to sign to get Pete eligible. Pete and I had already decided on our course of action. We never had any hesitation. She faxed the papers. I signed. We had formally applied to participate in a clinical trial.

By the end of that day, January 13, we had surgery scheduled for January 17 at the clinic. The catheter placement surgery for the IL-13 treatment was tentatively scheduled for January 26. All this was done in about two weeks from Pete's initial diagnosis.

The doctor sharing a prognosis and life expectancy estimate for Pete had both positive and negative effects. It helped us get a perspective on what we were facing. I remember at one point Dr. Barnett shared the positive, proven results when Temodar was administered with radiation (a standard practice for treatment of brain tumors). He seemed so enthusiastic to report that life expectancy was increased by three. I felt hopeful!

"Three what?" I asked. "Three times longer to live? Or by three years? Three what?"

Dr. Barnett looked at me a little surprised and matter-of-factly said "Three months."

My heart dropped into my stomach. He had talked with such promise about Temodar, and all that would give Pete was a lousy three months! That was why it was good to have doctors share prognosis information. They are in the business of saving lives at all costs. Sharing the prognosis information gave us the urgency to make the necessary decisions even in the face of such risk and impact.

The negative aspect of sharing a prognosis and estimate for life expectancy was the problem with all numbers. Pete and I knew the doctors were talking in averages. Pete wasn't an average; he was an individual, one single person. Those averages may or may not apply to him. He might live less than they estimated, or he might live longer, or he might be healed completely, because we knew God wasn't bound by doctors' estimates. So we found those kinds of estimates helpful to know, but we did not consider them truth. We did not know, nor did they, how Pete was going to respond to surgery or treatment.

From my prayer journal: January 11 and 12, 2006

Next step in this adventure today, Lord. We seek your wisdom. I have no idea where this adventure is leading us. May your sanctifying love redeem me and Pete in this circumstance. If this is the end of Pete's life as we know it—so be it. I accept that you will restore and make him whole in your life forever. If you see a mission for us here, then so be it, too. I dread the worst—Pete in a vegetable state and requiring care, but having no engagement with life. But whatever you will, Lord. We trust in you. Protect Pete from evil. Give him your strength. Your power. You are so dynamic—if your presence is with Pete, he will be a reflection of your life—dynamic-alive-changing-no matter what.

Pete's prognosis is terrifying but real. I know you are not bound by the prognosis of men. Can I have him for a little while longer? Bless us with your presence. We will treasure each day. I have such conflicting feelings. I want to hope and trust in your power, believe in your healing of Pete, and simultaneously help Pete prepare for his death and help him get ready. May your glory shine here, Lord!

5

Facing Death

Pete did not slip into depression. After the first shock of the life expectancy numbers, Pete never again talked about how long he had to live. He never showed anxiety. He did become sad, and more than anything else, he became easily touched by others' kindness. It was as if his heart was raw and exposed. Any action of kindness, regardless how small, would make his eyes grow misty with tears.

I think Pete moved fast in facing his own death. It was how he had dealt with any new truth or new fact in his life. He did this privately. He did it quickly. I'm almost sure I know when he did. I felt only respect and admiration for him.

Throughout New Year's weekend of 2005/2006, Pete carved out some time to be alone, while we were with our rowdy group of friends. This was very unusual for him. I never remembered Pete going off alone before in any setting, let alone during a visit with our friends. We were in South Carolina that weekend, spending New Year's in a friend's home with our Boston friends. We'd all be gathered in the kitchen or around the TV, and I'd look around and Pete would be gone. I'd find him upstairs away from the noise, reading a book he had received that Christmas, *Epic* by John Eldredge. This little pocket book was given to him by a Crossroads volunteer, leader, Missy, who we served with. The book was about the story of life. Eldredge's little book had four chapters and an epilogue. The chapters are titled Acts One through Four. Eldredge used the following quote to preface his book: "I had always felt life first as a story—and if there is a story there is a story teller" (G.K. Chesterton).

Pete pored over this book. He underlined many sentences. I think this book helped Pete come to terms with his own death. He faced death squarely and courageously. He faced his death with faith. Eldredge's book helped him do so. Here was what Pete underlined in this story.

> But now let us lift our eyes to the horizon and see what the future holds in store... God has set eternity in our hearts... This is written on the human heart, this longing for happily ever after. You see, every story has an ending. Every story, including yours. Have you ever faced this? Sooner or later, life will break your heart. Or rather, death will break your heart.
>
> This happy ending is borrowed right out of the Scripture. An immortal life. The restoration of all things. A wedding feast. In hope beyond hope, Paradise is regained. This is what God has been trying to say to us all along... The restoration of the world played out before us each spring and summer is precisely what God is promising us about our lives. Every miracle Jesus ever did was pointing to this Restoration. At the end of Act Three, he announces: 'I make all things new' (Rev 21:5)
>
> So we too shall live and never die. Creation will be restored... Imagine being reunited with the ones we love... We will walk with God in the Garden... There'll be wine at the Banquet.

Pete really liked the idea that there would be wine in heaven! We talked of this many times afterward. I heard the author talking to Pete:

> "Things are not what they seem, Pete. You must live as though the unseen world (the rest of reality) is weightier and more real and more dangerous than the part of reality we can see. This is a Love Story, set in the midst of a life-and-death battle. This is war—a battle for the human heart. You have a crucial role to play... We have reached the moment where we, too, must find our courage and rise up to recover our hearts and fight for the hearts of others. The hour is late, and much time wasted... May you play your part well."

The way Pete expressed his acceptance of his death and his trust in God was shown in the way he responded to me whenever we talked about future events that were giving me anxiety. I'd ask Pete things like: "Are you worried about surgery?" or "Are you concerned about what will happen after surgery?" or "Are you anxious about visiting the doctor today and what the MRI results will show?"

Pete would simply say, "We will have to just see what the Lord's plan is."

And that was it. The end of discussion.

Most mornings, Pete and I would pray before we ate breakfast. I would usually let Pete start the prayer. Each morning, he'd say, "Thanks, God, for letting me wake up! How thankful I am to have this day." Then he'd look at me and say, "And to have this day with you!"

My response to Pete's predicted short life expectancy was not to accept it. I understood the medical facts. I didn't deny the scientific basis behind the medical experts' assessment. I knew they thought Pete would die soon. I didn't think Pete was an exception. I just believed with all my heart in God's possible healing of Pete. No guarantee from God. Just a possibility.

In the face of Pete's death sentence, I studied every healing story in the Bible, and I prayed for Pete's healing every day. I believed God could heal Pete. The only question was, would He? Was Pete's healing part of his purpose for Pete and me?

"News about him spread all over Syria, and people brought to him all who were ill with various diseases, those suffering severe pain, the demon-possessed, those having seizures, and the paralyzed, and he healed them." (Matthew 4:24) I noted with special interest the number of healing stories in the Bible where someone other than the person needing healing made the request. I was the one asking for Pete's healing. I never heard Pete ask God for his own healing. Doesn't mean he didn't, but he never verbalized that to me. The prayers Pete shared with me were only full of thankfulness, appreciation and love. But no requests. So I was relieved to see how many times Jesus healed someone based on the request of another who loved them.

"Some men brought to Jesus a paralytic, lying on a mat. When Jesus saw their faith, he said to the paralytic, "Take heart son, your sins are forgiven... Get up, take your mat and go home." (Matthew 9: 2–7) This guy's friends were crazy. They couldn't get into the house where Jesus was because of the crowd, so they climbed up on the roof, cut a hole, and rappelled the guy down into the room where Jesus was. Jesus liked their faith. What was a little inconvenience like driving to Cleveland in the snow compared to that?

And there was this story: "There was a centurion's servant whom his master valued highly, was sick and about to die. The centurion heard of Jesus and sent some elders of the Jews to him asking him to come and heal his servant... He was not far from the house when the centurion sent friends to say to him, 'Lord don't trouble yourself, for I do not deserve to have you come under my roof... But say the word and my servant will be healed.' When Jesus heard this he was amazed." (Luke 7:2–9)

This story spoke to me. I thought of all the ways that I had failed in my life. I knew I didn't deserve God's mercy on Pete. What made me think Jesus would hear my request? The Roman soldier felt the same way. He wasn't Jewish. Jesus was a Jew, so he sent his Jewish friends to ask Jesus for him. I had asked many Christians far more spiritual than I to pray for Pete. "Ask for Pete and ask for me," I had said. Just "say the word," I begged Jesus. "That's all that was needed. Your word can heal Pete."

These Bible stories gave me hope. They made me determined to keep asking! I asked God for Pete's healing multiple times every day. I had asked again the day Pete died. I had asked for seven hundred and sixty-seven days.

From my prayer journal: January 2006

I ask you to heal and restore Pete. Get rid of this tumor and cancer. I know you are not bound by the prognosis of men. Your power is greater than any of us. I sense I may lose Pete, my friend for life. I feel blessed to have had his friendship for as long as I have. You give and You take away.

Can I love him for a little longer, please?

6

Enlisting an Army
of Supporters

Our first phone calls right after Christmas were to our two sons, Michael and Steve. Both were grown men and living away from Cincinnati—Michael in Florida, Steve in the Washington DC area. It was hard to communicate by phone news of such impact. We couldn't see their faces, or hug them, or be hugged by them, as the news sank in. Neither son was especially communicative about most things.

We spoke to Michael first. Pete and I would both get on the phone when we talked with either son. Michael was out walking his dog. I was not sure he understood the implications—or maybe he didn't want to. "I have a brain tumor," Pete said, tears in his eyes as the words tumbled out.

"Well, you can get better, can't you?" Michael asked his dad in a desperate tone of voice. "They can fix it, can't they?" Without waiting for an answer, he blurted out, "Then, get on with whatever it takes!"

Pete and I looked at each other after we hung up.

"I don't think he gets it," I said.

Pete just nodded. His eyes were full of sadness.

Our other son, Steve, was hunting in West Virginia. We talked with our daughter-in-law Kathy, and explained Pete's news. She was

35

stunned and very quiet. We knew she'd find a way to get to Steve. We connected with Steve briefly later that night from his favorite diner. The cell connection was very poor, and we had a hard time hearing each other.

"We will talk more when you get home," Pete told Steve.

We both knew Michael and Steve would call each other shortly and trade notes.

Our relationship with both sons deepened significantly during Pete's illness. Both sons got more engaged with their father and with me, not less. They did not step away from us, but stepped toward us. Steve was on a plane to Cincinnati from Washington DC shortly after we got back from our New Year's trip. It was a few days before we headed to the Cleveland Clinic to get a second opinion. He and his dad did his dad's to-do list. Pete felt such an urgency to get the house ready for me, in case anything happened to him during surgery. Pete was so happy working next to his son. They cleaned gutters, fixed the stereo, and set up the TV. They changed light bulbs, and set up automatic lights for security purposes. They worked for days side by side, with lots of trips to Home Depot, and fun dinners at Steve's favorite Cincinnati restaurants at night. Pete was so happy. I felt such comfort just having Steve there. Phone calls between Steve and his dad began almost daily from then on. Steve rarely missed a day calling his dad, unless he was traveling out of the country.

Michael was more silent, but not less feeling. He made trips home, too, and due to the timing of his trips, shared care-giving duties with me more than Steve did. Pete had been very sick almost each time Michael visited. On one trip, he helped me get Pete to his radiation treatments, almost carrying his father into the car. He fed his dad when Pete wouldn't eat. Pete ate for Michael when he wouldn't eat for anyone else. Michael is an expert chef. He made his dad a dinner of all dinners on one of his trips home. I had never seen such love poured into a meal. Michael was with us during mini-crises. He responded with compassion, and urgency, and good practical sense. It was like having the best of his healthy Dad with me.

The day after talking to the guys, Pete and I were on a plane headed to Charleston, South Carolina to spend New Year's Eve with four friends. We had a New Year's Eve tradition over the last fifteen years of spending New Year's in a different city every year with the same good friends. We had been in Cleveland and Boston and Tampa and Chicago and West Palm and London. This year it was Charleston! That afternoon at the hotel bar, Pete practiced telling friends for the first time in person. Pete cried easily when telling others his diagnosis. Not a sobbing cry—just tears welling up in his eyes. I can remember our friend Judith's reaction the best: "You are going to be okay, Pete. I just know it." Her bold confidence was a comfort to me often over the coming months. I remembered her unbridled confidence in Pete's recovery again and again when things felt so hopeless. Of all the hundred of friends and associates and family members we told about Pete's situation, there were only two people, one being Judith, who expressed such unwavering confidence in Pete's recovery.

I began telling the rest of my family members and my associates at work about Pete's situation. Pete did the same at his business and with some clients. I can remember my sister-in-law Paula's conversation with me. She is a practicing nurse.

"A brain tumor," she said. "A GBM. Oh, Kathy. That's real bad. I mean really bad. Oh, I can't believe it," she said, holding back tears.

The positive aspect of telling others, for me, was making it real. Friends and family like Paula helped me realize it was real. I wasn't watching a movie. I cried with Paula on the phone.

Pete called two of his best friends, and while telling them his diagnosis and next steps for treatment, asked them if they would be pallbearers for him at his funeral! Jerry, Pete's best friend from Tampa, recalled almost swerving off the road, since Pete caught him on his cell phone while he was driving home from work.

Pete told Dave and the rest of the Angus Group staff that same week. He fought through tears. A man who had rarely cried in private was now full of emotion in public whenever he spoke of his diagnosis. Sadness filled him. He was saying goodbye each time he shared his news.

I told the individuals who reported to me at the bank about Pete's diagnosis. I told them that I would be leaving work, and I was not sure when I would return. I told them that I saw this chance to be a caregiver for Pete as a "lucky chance" for me. I was "lucky" because I now had the chance to return a little of the care Pete had given me for the last twenty years as my partner. He had done so many things to support me in my career. I felt blessed to have the chance to give a little of that back to him. I used to laugh when I told him, "I could take care of you for the next ten years, and still not put a dent in what I owed you for all the times you took care of me and supported my success for the last twenty!"

I was lucky because the bank had been so generous to me and Pete that I didn't have the financial pressure many have in trying to be a caregiver and work at the same time. I didn't have those tensions. I was lucky because Pete and I had a chance to love each other now in an even more intimate way than ever before. Every day we would be together. We had never experienced that before in our twenty-plus years of marriage!

I had all my managers who reported to me, as well as our key business partners together, in Phoenix on January 3, 2006 for a couple of days to complete our annual planning. I was surprised that I cried as hard as I did when I told my team about Pete's brain tumor and his prognosis. I told them I would be gone most of the first quarter, and wasn't sure when I would return. I knew that they would all step up. I told them who would be in charge while I was gone. They were quiet, and many cried with me.

In between the tears I told them, "I feel lucky. I now have a chance to give back to Pete a little of the care he has given to me over the last twenty years, as I built my career at the bank." I told them what I had told Pete. "I could care for Pete for the next ten years, and still not put a dent in what I owed him for all the times he took care of me over the last twenty. I know you know how special of a partner Pete has been for me. I could never have done what I did for our company without him."

Before we left Phoenix, my team did a beautiful thing for me. Earlier in the day one of my regional managers had asked me to stop up to his hotel room, so his wife and he could pray with me. That was a first for me. I had never prayed before with a fellow worker. They prayed for Pete's healing. They asked God to give me strength, and asked God to be present with us both on our journey ahead. Already, Pete's circumstance was changing things.

Then, at the end of our planning meeting, the whole team circled around me and shared with me all the ways they appreciated who I was as their leader and as their friend. Each person spoke from their heart. I was moved. I felt so loved and so supported. What a gift they gave me! It was as if they were preparing me with the necessary armor to do battle. God had shown up.

My former boss, Richard, who was now president of the bank and a good friend, had asked me if Pete and I had talked yet to our pastor at our church. Richard and I had known each other for over ten years. He knew and loved Pete, too. We hadn't even thought about talking to a pastor. We didn't really have traditional pastors at Crossroads, but I distinctly felt God's hand leading me through Richard's suggestion. I asked one of our volunteer leaders, and was directed to Steve Mercer, who was the Director of Pastoral Care at Crossroads. He agreed to meet with us. Pete and I went out to visit him one cold January afternoon right before we were scheduled to leave for the Cleveland Clinic for Pete's surgery. Steve was wonderful, kind and caring and practical. He pointed to a "Be Bold" sign on his white board in his office, and told us, "Be bold with God. Ask for what you want from Him with confidence." I remembered Steve's advice. Over and over again I would say to myself when things looked bad. "Be bold with God. Ask with confidence!"

We told Steve we were going to the Cleveland Clinic for probably the better part of the next three months. Earlier that very day, Steve had met with a representative from Carepages, and was about to engage Crossroads in a partnership with them. He told us this was a great service. We might want to use it, since we were going to be separated from many family members and friends. Carepages was a free web site service which would allow us to communicate and keep in contact with all. I remember thinking, ugh! A web page. I groaned. I didn't have much confidence about setting up a web page. My employees used to describe me as technologically handicapped.

We actually set the Carepage web site up in the car on the drive to Cleveland that Sunday before surgery. "Pete's Carepage!" it was titled. It was that easy! It was a fantastic tool for us. We would provide updates on Pete's condition through this website, and everyone who was following Pete could also send us messages, and they could read each others' messages as well as our updates. How cool was that! Once our Carepage was set up, we notified all possible interested persons that the site was live, and gave them instructions on how they could access it. Mike did lots of this notification for us by email to friends, family and business associates. Once we let a critical mass know, they spread the word to others. The Carepage was a HUGE source of support for me as a caregiver and for Pete. From January 15, 2006 until January 26, 2008 we had over twenty-six thousand hits to that site, and over eight hundred people following us from all over the country. Here's how we started Pete's page.

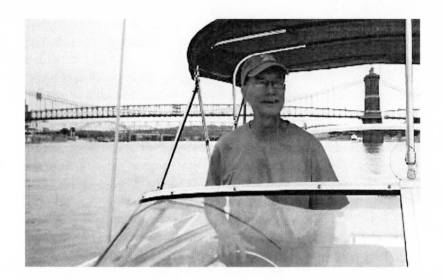

PETE CAPTAINING HIS BOAT, "MY DESTINATION"

January 15, 2006 at 04:16 p.m.

Welcome to Pete's Carepage! This will be our primary way of keeping everyone informed on how Pete and Kathy are doing. The following backdated updates are to give everyone the chain of events that led Pete to Cleveland for surgery on Tuesday. In addition to reading updates about Pete, you can send messages to Pete and Kathy on this site. We will let you know what time surgery will be as soon as we know ourselves. Thanks for your prayers and support.

§ § § § §

A message from Craig and Barbara Wolf

Craig Wolf January 15, 2006 at 05:15 PM EST

Pete and Kathy—We are shocked by this news of what you're going through, but encouraged, as you must be, by the superb team of doctors you have on your side. As you know, we are all too aware of how fragile life can be, and we know that prayer works! Please know that you have our prayers with you, and especially on Tuesday for the surgery. We will keep in touch through this message board.

All our best, Craig and Barbara

§ § § § §

The Carepage site was an invaluable tool to me and Pete. I updated our Carepage frequently, and I was honest with our readers. They knew most of what Pete and I and the family knew. This transparency made others feel really connected to us in a genuine way. In addition to providing information to all those interested, I used the Carepage to ask for prayer requests. "This is what Pete needs now," I would write. I had been taught to pray for specific requests, and I soon became very dependent on this form of communication. When we got a piece of bad news, or Pete's condition deteriorated, I'd jump on the Carepages, because I wanted all those hundreds of people storming the heavens for us!

Needless to say, Pete had colleagues, friends and business associates all over the country, as did I. Instead of repeating over and over the same update information, I could update once, and all those who wanted to know could know our situation by accessing the website. On their email they'd get a message as soon as I posted an update: "Pete Nadherny Carepage has been updated." I was told that at the bank, an updated message on Pete's Carepage was hot news, and employees would race to share our news with each other.

Pete and I never really talked about whether we wanted to share the details of his situation with others. We just did it. Some may be much more hesitant to be as transparent with others as we were. We felt that we were in such a desperate situation; we needed all the support we could muster from others.

I have since discovered that there is another website called Lotsahelpinghands.com, which can actually request and schedule services others are willing to provide: visiting times, food drop-offs, errands that needed to be run, children's pick-up times and more. It's another wonderful tool I would have used if I had known about it then.

The Crossroads community was in itself its own army of supporters for Pete and me. On Sunday, January 15' the Crossroads community offered to hold a prayer service for us before we left for surgery at the clinic. The reading that morning at the service was Jeremiah 29:11. "For I know the plans I have for you... plans to prosper you and not to harm you, plans to give you a hope and a future." I cried during the reading, so touched by the message. How much more encouragement could God have given to us?

I can still see all the faces that came to our prayer service. The room was full of both adults and children. My dad had his hand on Pete's shoulder. Our Senior Pastor, Brian, held Pete's hand and kneeled in front of him. Jerry, a Crossroads Elder, led the prayer service for us. Friends were present. Community members from our Crossroads ministry teams were there. There must have been eighty or so believers gathered for Pete and me. Pete was overwhelmed by this show of support. He closed his eyes and bowed his head. They laid hands on both of us, and anointed us with oil to give us strength. We were reminded to be relentless with God, asking persistently for Pete's healing, just like the widow had asked the judge relentlessly. We both felt humbled, and full of gratitude. Without going back home, Pete and I climbed in our car. We were off to Cleveland! Pete drove. It didn't snow. Mike and Mary Jo were right behind us in their car all the way up.

The greatest comfort to Pete and to me was the commitment Mary Jo and Mike made to Pete and me. They were the first people Pete called to tell them what his full-body scan had revealed. They kept our secret with us until after Christmas. Mike had just retired from his post-retirement job as the president of a school, so his time had not been redistributed to others yet. Mary Jo was working part-time as a minister to the sick and elderly in a Catholic parish. They were able to devote their time to us, and they chose to do so! They went with us to doctor visits. They stayed with us for both surgeries in Cleveland. Their kids came to Cleveland to visit Pete in the hospital. Mary Jo had medical knowledge that I would rely on hundreds of times when I was fearful, or wanted a second opinion on a symptom.

Mike and Pete became like brothers, and Pete would share with Mike feelings that he would not even share with me. He could complain about me to Mike, and share his deepest sadness and distress without fear of upsetting Mike. Mike and Pete found out they liked many of the same things: wine, cars, women, salmon, and vanilla ice cream drizzled with chocolate syrup. They laughed together all the time, deep belly laughs like boys do in junior high.

One night when we went out to dinner before we left for Cleveland, Mary Jo and Mike told us, "We are committed to join you on this journey. We will walk with you every step of the way. No one should have to make this journey alone." And they did. And they have. Sometimes God sends angels.

I am almost embarrassed about the support Pete and I received during our journey. I had an understanding employer who let me take as much leave as I needed to care for Pete, no questions asked. Pete had a business partner who could have pulled the terms of their contract, that would have forced a sale of Pete's share in the business, but he did not. We had a church community that reached out and enclosed us in their arms. We had supportive family members, many of whom knew something about medicine! We had friends, lots of them, willing to help. Their cards and letters and gifts filled our home. One bank colleague knitted a shawl for Pete to keep him warm, saying prayers continually for him as she knit. Another group actually sent a prayer shawl. Pete got his favorite sausages sent from Chicago's Portillo's. Homemade soups and meals filled our freezer.

I learned to be specific in my asking for help. I was ready when someone offered. I had a list of needs always by the phone, so when help was offered, I could be specific in the way someone could help. Firewood was one example. Pete had always brought home firewood for our fireplace. We didn't have enough to make it through the winter. I knew I could not handle that task alone.

Nora asked, "How can I help?"

I was ready. "Do you have a wood-burning fireplace?" I asked.

"Yes," she said.

"Do you know anyone who delivers firewood?" She did not know of anyone, but within a week, there Nora and Tom were at our door with a truckload of firewood to unload. They told me later how much comfort it gave them to think of Pete sitting in his chair on a cold Ohio winter's night knowing a fire would be burning making us cozy, thanks to them.

Children. Family members. Friends. Business associates. Church community. Neighbors. Pete was by nature a rather conservative, private person. Now here we were, letting people into our lives and hearts faster than we had ever done before. We felt exposed. Nothing was private. We shared intimate details of our life. I don't know why we changed so fast. But we did. Perhaps it was God's way of answering our prayers and providing us comfort. For the first time in my life, I started to really believe in angels.

From my prayer journal: January 2006

I focus on your abundance. Your power. Your love for us. I trust in your love. Thank you for Craig, Crossroads, Nan and Bill, Mary Jo and Mike, Michael and Christine and Meg, Mom and Dad, Nora and Tom and all those others who are helping us. How grateful we are for them!

7

Surgery 1: Brain Tumor Removal

"The major goals of brain surgery are to:

Preserve or improve neurological function.

Obtain a piece of the tumor to confirm diagnosis (biopsy).

Remove the tumor completely or partially.

Insert a shunt, if needed to drain fluid or relieve pressure on the brain.

Implant chemotherapy wafers when needed.

Most studies have shown that the more tumor tissue that is removed, the better the survival rate and sometimes the quality of life."

−Brain Tumors: Finding the Ark.

There are a lot of different kinds of brain tumors and grades of brain tumors. A full listing and description can be found on the American Brain Tumor Association's website, as well as in many of the medical survival guides. The symptoms and the treatment for brain tumors are dependent on the type of tumor and location. Tumors in different parts of the brain affect different areas of function, thereby creating different symptoms and requiring different treatment plans.

Pete's tumor was a glioblastoma multiforme (GBM) grade IV in the left temporal lobe of his brain. A tumor in the temporal lobe affected hearing, language and memory. Memory, in the left temporal lobe, was affected in words and names. Pete couldn't remember his clients' names—that was his first symptom! Later, any word that had a capital letter became impossible for Pete to recall. Didn't matter if it was a person's name or a city or a state or a country. Pete stopped calling me or his sons by name. If Pete's tumor had been in his right temporal lobe instead of the left, he would have had memory problems, but it would have shown up in not recalling pictures or faces. Pete always recognized us; he just couldn't find our names. If Pete's tumor had been in the frontal lobe instead of the temporal lobe, he might have had personality changes, a problem concentrating or mobility issues instead of memory and speech challenges.

Brain cells can't regenerate. Once a brain tumor has killed cells and/or injured surrounding tissue, they can't grow back. Pete's tumor was fast-growing. Before he ever had surgery, the cells in his brain that enabled him to remember names had been destroyed. They would never come back. And as the tumor grew or if it recurred, damaged tissue from surgery or other treatment affected his functionality in a definitive way. Brain cancer is a cruel disease.

Pete's surgery was scheduled for Tuesday January 17, 2006. We were driving to Cleveland on Sunday, January 15, because January 16 was a full day of surgery preparation at the clinic. Saturday night, January 14, was Pete's and my last night at home. We usually marked special occasions by going out to eat, so that is what we did: dinner at the best steakhouse in Cincinnati with our favorite bottle of wine— just the two of us. That night Pete started a journal, although I am stretching the definition of a journal by calling it that. Pete would not have called it a journal. He didn't really like to write, and had never written except when he had to. But he started writing in a pocket-sized notebook that night! I never knew he had done this. He had never shared it with me. I found it in his nightstand later. In his notebook, he made eight entries. They are precious to me.

Jan 14, 2006—Cincinnati Saturday (Pete's Journal)

THE Planning is over. What planning, Kathy! Wow! Her family and friends. Absolutely perfect dinner at the Precinct given as a birthday present to me from her family. Kathy is wonderful! Take charge. Plan. Attitude. Thoughts with God.

Bill & Nan.

All the friends. Emails. Cards. Love, prayers.

Yet—Surreal?

God, I am with you.

On that Sunday, January 15, after the prayer service at Crossroads, Pete drove me to Cleveland, with Mike and Mary Jo in their car right behind us. We got settled in our hotel room by late afternoon. Each time we traveled to Cleveland for Pete's medical care, we would try to make it fun. Pete loved to eat out, and Cleveland had some outstanding restaurants. I had received lots of referrals from my bank team in that market. The first choice this trip was Italian, Pete's favorite kind of food. We went to Johnny's in Cleveland with Mary Jo, Mike, Steve and his wife, Kathy, who had flown from Washington D.C. just in time to join us. And what a time we had. Lots of wine!

Jan 15, 2006—Cleveland Sunday (Pete's Journal)

Church with Dad, Caleb, Michaela, Mike, Mary Jo, Shauna, Kathy. WOW! And what a service. Appropriate plus++ Then all the friends—praying with us before the service. Brian, Family, Friends. How do you describe? Thanks God! Incredible. Hands. Feelings. Love, Prayers.

Great for Kathy, too. Better than expected for her!

So I got to drive. The whole way to Cleveland. Thanks.

Kathy, Steve, Kathy-Perfect! What a GREAT family!

And all the calls to the car. Driving with music from our neighbor, Dianne.

Then dinner with Mike and Mary Jo also and Steve's ordering (the wine) Plumpjack! WOW!

God thanks.

Swept the deck in Cincinnati!

On Monday morning, January 16, we started the day at the Brain Tumor Institute. The Cleveland Clinic was six blocks long. Each building was named by a letter. "R" was the Brain Tumor Institute; "L" was the building where we got the MRI.

On the day before surgery, Dr. Barnett's assistant, Gail, stuck lime-green markers on Pete's head to help Dr. Barnett locate the right places to operate, using the microscopic brain surgery technique he had mastered. Pete built his own chart in order to get admitted to the clinic. Chart in hand, he walked from one building to the next, completing the necessary paperwork. It took all day: the blood labs, MRI scan, admissions, insurance. It was a little overwhelming, but a very efficient system. We didn't have to wait long anywhere. We all noticed how kind all the staff were. Pete was exhausted from all the walking—where he went, his entourage of the five of us would follow, his chart getting bigger after every stop.

Dinner that night before surgery was in Little Italy. Michael was now in from Florida, shivering in Cleveland's thirty-degree temperatures. Pete wore a knit hat to cover the lime green markers that looked like Life Savers on his head. What a funny group we were. We laughed and laughed during dinner. Michael cried, as he hugged his father goodnight back at the hotel.

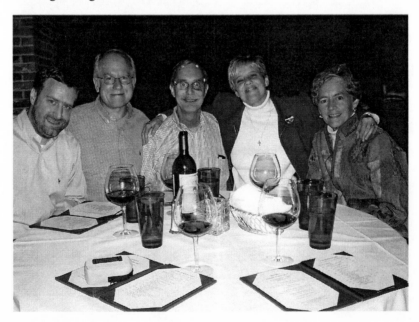

Steve, Mike, Pete, Mary Jo and Kathy—the night before surgery

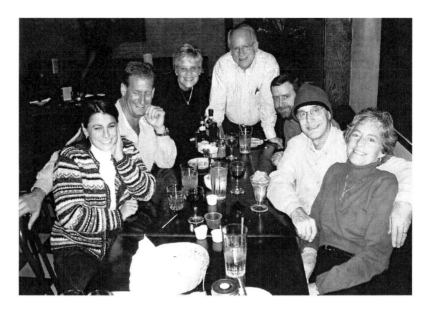

Kathy, Michael, Mary Jo, Mike, Steve, Pete, and Kathy

We were back in the hotel room and I was exhausted, and I wasn't the one with the brain tumor! Pete was sitting in a chair by the TV.

"What are you doing?' I asked. "Come get into bed. It's late."

He said, "I am writing out notes to a few people, in case I don't make it out of surgery tomorrow. I want you to distribute them when the time is right."

I was stunned. Between my tiredness and my surprise, I just looked at him so tenderly, got out of bed and put my arms around him. I was silent. I had no need to reassure him of his safety the next day. He knew all that I knew.

This was a sacred moment. Pete had met death in the face, and he wasn't afraid. He just wanted to make sure he had a chance to say good-bye to a few special people just in case. Pete being his cautious self, and realistic about the risks, had written good-bye notes to Steven, Michael, Mike and Mary Jo, Dave, his business partner, and me. After he finished, he put them in a small box, and placed them in his duffel bag.

January 16, 2006, Monday—Cleveland (Pete's journal)

Tests today. Michael joins. Writing hard notes. Getting ready for Tuesday. All Day! Dinner at Trattoria's on the Hill. Great Italian.

Mike & Mary Jo, Mike's helping with dessert—How Nice ...

They say "No" to the condo for us. Makes sense. Kathy can work downtown.

Steve is the 'Stone.' Really helpful. (His) Kathy is fun with Steve and holding up Michael. I missed it. Michael is out of it. The pressure. WOW!

And my Kathy—loving, perfect as always!!

Counting down.

January 17—Cleveland, Tuesday (Pete's journal)

Today is the day. Probably no notes for awhile... God, I'm in your hands. I will take one, just one big angel though.

From my prayer journal: January 17, 2006—Cleveland Clinic, Pete's surgery

Thanks, Lord, for all the gifts and prayers and love you have given Pete and I. The support of family. Your love is evident. May I love Pete as you would love him today. May I be full of comfort for him. May I be a confident presence. Eliminate all of our fear. Be present today. Guide Dr. Barnett's hand and his judgment. Make it your hand and your wisdom. Get rid of this tumor today and eliminate all those cancer cells that surround the tumor. I love you. You have precious Pete in your hands today. Send your words of comfort to him during his surgery and as he recovers. Amen.

Pete and I, Steve, Michael, and Kathy walked over to the Cleveland Clinic's Surgery center—Building E. Pete reported in at 9:30 a.m. Mary Jo and Mike joined us there. This was a huge space. The reception desk was the center of activity. Dr. Barnett said surgery would last four to six hours. Pete got into pre-op by 10:15 a.m., which meant he took off his street clothes, got into a hospital gown, and the nurses did the last lab tests and checks. We stayed with him, all of us crowding into a little cubicle with curtains around this big circular nursing station. A bank friend stopped by, knowing exactly where we would be, since her brother was a brain tumor survivor, and she had been in this very room a few years ago. Mary Ellen. How comforting she was. She touched us and then left us, respecting those private moments only family can share.

Pete and I got some time alone. We held hands. I looked in his eyes and he looked back into mine. My eyes went to his wedding ring, which he kept on. We cried. "I love you," He said.

"And I love you," was all I remember us saying. Steve, Kathy, Michael, Mary Jo and Mike came in and joined us, circling Pete, who was on a stretcher. We prayed together. We asked for Michael the Archangel to show his power, be Pete's warrior and do battle for Pete.

And sure enough, that big angel Pete had asked God for, appeared. The orderly who was to take Pete into the operating room heard us praying outside the curtain. He stuck his head in. He grinned. "I'm Chris," he said. He prayed with us. Then as he wheeled Pete away he said over his shoulder, "I'll pray Pete right into surgery." What a gift. I left Pete in Chris' hands.

The Surgery Center had TV-type screens that monitored a patient's progress throughout surgery. It reminded me of those screens at airports that tell you if the plane is at the gate or if boarding has started. We could tell Pete Nadherny was in surgical prep at 11:15 a.m. His initials, "Na... Y.P," printed on the screen just this way. It was like his flight number, and told us the progress of his surgery. Surgery actually didn't start until 1:30 p.m. Gail called and told us that getting the computer right for the surgery took longer than Dr. Barnett had expected. We got a call at 3:30 and again at 4:30 p.m., letting us know that things were going according to plan. Pete's vital signs were good, meaning his body was handling the surgery trauma well. They told us there was still a long way to go.

I couldn't begin to count the number of times Mary Jo walked up and stared at that TV screen, looking and hoping for updates on Pete. Worrying with me was what sisters did. She was a great sister to me. Time crawled. Michael slept. Steve worked on his computer, remodeling his house. I read. Mike and Mary Jo walked the floor, and talked on their cell phone to family back at home. Seemed forever.

At around seven p.m., we started getting hungry. The surgery center had gotten eerily quiet. The screen read "Na... Y.P was in PACU (Post-Anesthesiology Care Unit) at 18:47 p.m." That meant the surgery was over. Pete was in recovery.

At 7:46 the receptionist said, "The doctor is on the phone for you.

I was shaking a little. I had yellow post-it notes and a pen in my hand. Mary Jo was right next to me.

Dr. Barnett said "All's done. Pete's in the process of waking up. He had a seizure in the tongue and face as we were moving him into recovery. Took us a while to figure out he was having a seizure." I could hear tenseness in Dr. Barnett's voice. He continued: "I am not leaving the hospital until I get the results of the CAT scan. Sent Pete for the scan now. I want to make sure Pete isn't bleeding. It might have been the Keppra; the anti-seizure medication wasn't strong enough to hold through the surgery. I have given Pete a strong dose of Atavan and Dilantin to calm him down."

I went back and reported to the guys and Mike. I was shaking from fear and exhaustion. We were all quiet.

By 8:15 Dr. Barnett called back to tell me there was no bleeding. He was going home. I was relieved. I could hear the relief in his voice. The hospital staff would call me later, and tell me when we could come down and see Pete.

More waiting. By now we were very hungry, so Michael and Steve and Mike decided to make a food run. Subway and McDonald's closed at nine o'clock. As they were on the run, we got the call that we could come down to recovery. They got the food and met us in recovery.

The recovery room was in the basement. We arrived and they wouldn't let us in. We looked around. Gray linoleum floors and long white walls. There were two lonely orange plastic chairs in the hall. The rest of us sat on the floor. We looked like refugees eating our sandwiches, and waiting for the word that we could get in to see Pete. We were all pretty quiet. We watched hospital staff in scrubs taking mysterious-looking substances through the pathology doors right next to us.

It was after ten p.m. when we got to see Pete. He looked awful. He looked yellow. The left side of his head was bandaged with white gauze about two inches wide, which ran from the center of his head following his hairline to just above his ear. IV tubes were everywhere. He was sleepy, restless and very confused. He couldn't open his eyes, but was moving his body around in awkward starts. He did not speak.

Pete's Carepage: January 18, 2006, 12:32 a.m.

We are now on the neurology ICU floor, which means Pete is finally coming out of recovery. Pete is conscious at moments but heavily sedated. All vital signs are good although he can't speak yet. It's been a long day but reading all of your messages and seeing all of

your names on our Carepage lifts my spirits and gives me strength.
How can we thank you enough for all the support? God is good and
we are lucky.

We found out much later that Pete had nearly died in recovery. He
had a status seizure that lasted for almost twenty minutes. Most seizures last a maximum of two to three minutes. Dr. Barnett told me he
thought the anti-seizure medication, Keppra, wasn't strong enough to
hold during the trauma of surgery. He blasted Pete with drugs, Atavan
and Dilantin, to get the seizure to stop. All the operating room staff
was nervous that this happened. The drugs were going to make Pete's
recovery time slower.

Mary Jo and Mike volunteered to stay the night with Pete. I was so
grateful for their offer! I was exhausted and almost numb. It was two
a.m. now, and I wanted to be back early in the morning to see the doctor. I walked across the street to the hotel, and fell asleep like I was
drugged.

Mike was next to Pete's bed when Pete got agitated and woke
around 4:30 a.m. Mike could tell Pete wanted to know what happened, but couldn't speak to ask. Mike said he put himself in Pete's
place, and figured he would answer the questions he would have had
if he was Pete.

Mike told him, "The tumor is gone. Dr Barnett got ninety-nine percent of it out. You did well. Your speech should start coming back in
the next few days."

Pete relaxed with Mike's presence. Mike drew a picture for Pete of
the tumor being ninety-nine percent gone. Mike and Pete bonded at
that moment. They became brothers. Pete fell back to sleep.

The next morning I was at the hospital at 6:30. Pete was in the
Neurology-ICU Step Down unit. He was sleeping when I arrived.
Mary Jo & Mike were sleeping in the waiting room around the corner.
I sent them home after they told me about Pete's reaction to Mike at
4:30 a.m. The step-down unit was a semi-circular room without walls.
Patients were separated by drawn curtains to create a cubicle. The
nursing station was against the wall in the middle of the semi-circle.
There was a small waiting room around the corner from the unit.

I started a daily routine of checking on Pete as soon as I arrived.
Most of the time he was still sleeping. I'd sit next to him and watch
him sleep. Touched his hand. The night nurses would let me into see
him, but didn't like me to stay when they were changing shifts. They
did an oral report, which could be heard by anyone in the patient cubi-

cles. So I'd leave Pete's cubicle when they started their report, and go around the corner to the waiting room. I would pray. I'd write my conversation with God in my journal, and read from the Bible. I was usually alone. It was a peaceful half-hour for me. I'd then go back to Pete's cubicle after shift change.

Dr. Barnett came in twice to see Pete the day after surgery. Barnett confirmed: "I got ninety-nine percent of the tumor out. It had grown since the last scan was taken. It was growing toward the back of the skull, and it will grow back if there is no treatment. The MRI looks great. No structure damage. Nothing is showing up except the empty space where the tumor was."

Dr. Barnett took a breath and quickly continued. "The seizure of the tongue was not identified right away. We were able to stop it, but it causes fatigue. The seizures overloaded Pete's circuits. I can't see any damage now, and am cautiously optimistic that Pete's speech will come back, like he was before the surgery. I was nowhere close to the speech/tongue center, so I still don't know what triggered the seizure. I was closest to the understanding part of the brain, and Pete's understanding is doing great."

To confirm that, Dr. Barnett would say to Pete, "Raise two fingers on your right hand," and Pete understood and executed his command. "I'm not sure now whether Pete will qualify for the IL-13 clinical trial. I have two weeks to make that decision. Let's get him recovered, and not have any more seizures. It didn't go as smoothly as planned," Barnett said, looking at me with an apology in his eyes.

I was pleased that Dr Barnett was able to get ninety-nine percent of the tumor out. That was better than I had expected. I was so relieved, because I knew Pete's life expectancy, and quality of life would be affected in a positive way. Dr. Barnett was apologetic for the seizure. I was just grateful for his competence, and caring for Pete. I don't know how much of the conversation with Dr. Barnett Pete understood. He was alert when Dr. Barnett spoke to him, as well as to me. But because Pete couldn't speak, I didn't know. As Pete gave a thumbs-up to the doctor as he left, I knew Pete was grateful, too. But a new worry arose for me: what if Pete couldn't qualify for the IL-13 clinical trial?

Each hour that first day, Pete was getting better. He was rolling his eyes at us when we said something he thought was stupid. He was in good spirits. By late afternoon, he could express himself pretty well. I could understand everything he was saying, compared to not understanding a word in the early morning. We could tell his thought processes were working. At first there were only words, then phrases, and by the end of the day, full sentences. The speech therapist came in and said he was doing well. She was very optimistic that Pete would return to full function. I felt relief. Leaky tears came over and over as Pete kept improving.

Pete was eating like a man who hadn't had food for days. Steve and Kathy smuggled into ICU a Wendy's chocolate Frosty, which he polished off after a complete dinner of chicken, mashed potatoes, gravy and ice cream. Pete was on twenty-four mgs. of dexamethosone (steroids), which I later came to understand was a huge dose. The steroids controlled the swelling in Pete's brain. One side effect was a voracious appetite.

That first day after surgery, we had our laptops in the cubicle in ICU, and Pete could read the messages streaming in to him from all over the country on his Carepage: family members, friends, business associates, all the bank people, and our friends at Crossroads. He smiled big at all those messages. He felt overwhelmed with the thought of responding to all of them.

"They are not expecting a reply," we said. Pete believed us, relief in his eyes.

By early evening he kept telling us, "I want you all to go out and have a big, nice dinner." He must have repeated it ten times or more. The thought of inconveniencing us was worrying him.

Mike, Mary Jo and Michael all laughed at him. "You're not getting rid of us that easy. Dinner at the cafeteria is just fine for us tonight!"

By the second day after surgery, the light was switched on in Pete's speech center. He was chatting away, got up to shave himself, went off pain medication, and other than a very nasty black left eye, Pete looked good.

"The black eye is normal," the nurses told us. "The blood drains there from the surgery, since it is the lowest place, and that causes the swelling." I sure wish someone had mentioned that before the surgery, as I was alarmed by the ugliness of his eye. "As the blood is absorbed, the swelling and discoloration will disappear," the nurses assured us.

The doctor ordered another EEG (electroencephalograph), which measures the electrical activity in the brain. The results were normal, showing no other seizure activity.

Dr. Barnett was pleased with Pete's progress. "We got this thing on the run now!" he said almost gleefully, like a soldier winning a battle.

Lack of memory was the most evident side effect of the surgery in Pete. The hospital put Pete through a series of questions about every four hours, to assess his mental state. He got a score. That same test would be used later to determine whether Pete was going to be eligible for the IL-13 clinical trial. All of us family members knew all the questions by heart now, and the repetition was numbing.

"Follow my finger," the nurse would say as she went right to left, and up and down past Pete's eyes. "Touch your index finger to your nose." "Tell me your name." "What is the date? Where are you right now? Who is the President of the United States?"

Pete, who was an avid Republican, couldn't remember that George W. Bush was president. We got a chuckle imagining our democratic family members, who loved to debate with Pete, knowing that in Pete's darkest moment, W. had abandoned him!

Pete was able to give his own name, and touch his nose with no problem. The date was more of a challenge, but he got it right after a few tries. But he could not say where he was. He couldn't find the answer "hospital," or the Cleveland Clinic, for any of the tests. We tried everything! We were playing charades with Pete behind the nurse, trying to give him hints. We played like our life depended on Pete's success in answering, and we pointed to every sign/cup/piece of memorabilia given him by the hospital to help him get it right. Nothing worked. Pete could not name the Cleveland Clinic as his current location. He couldn't even get out the word "hospital"—hotel was the closest he could come. Since I didn't know how this test would be scored, I fretted. What if Pete is not scoring high enough to become eligible for the clinical trial?

By the end of the second day, Pete had been moved out of the ICU Step-down unit, and was on a regular neurology floor. I was having normal conversations with him. He started taking long strolls around the hospital floor. He called his office, and was excited that one of his placements had closed while he was here.

"Making money even while staying at the Cleveland Clinic," Michael exclaimed. How delighted Pete was. His worry now was about the battery in the car. "What if it failed during our trips up and back in the harsh winter in Cleveland?" he asked. "We need to get a new one just in case."

My worry was about his eligibility for the clinical trial-IL-13. No assessment would be made until he returned next week, and they would see how he tested.

The surgical dressing was taken off the morning we headed home, Friday, January 20, 2006. There was an incision about six inches long from the crown of his head on the left side to right below his ear. There were over twenty sutures.

Pete called me on his cell phone about eight o'clock the night before we left the hospital. I was with the family in the hospital cafeteria getting dinner. "Where are my jeans? Did you steal my jeans?" he desperately asked.

"What do you need your jeans for?" I answered.

"I am getting ready to go home, and I can't find my jeans anywhere!" He had woken up from a sound sleep, and thought it was eight the next morning, and that I had stolen his jeans! Pete gave us all a needed laugh.

The day Pete left the hospital, he mastered where he was, the date and the day of the week. I felt some relief and thought maybe we would pass the eligibility test for the IL-13 study after all.

This man, Pete Nadherny, was amazing. Brain surgery on Tuesday. Home by Friday. Two-mile walks around our hilly neighborhood Mount Adams on Saturday and Sunday. Went to church. Did grocery shopping. Cooked steaks on the grill. Took me out to dinner one night. And surgery was less than a week before! Little did I know those would be the last walks we ever took around our neighborhood.

January 21, 2006—Cincinnati—Saturday (Pete's Journal)

At home! Wow. Missed the last few days after the surgery. The brain surgery started late and went really long. But I survived. Thanks God.

We drove home yesterday. I slept all the way.

What great help. Thank you Lord.

Mike & Steve called today. Kathy and I took a walk.

Lord, tomorrow is church. I'm ready. Next week to Cleveland again.

Mom & Dad will stop by tomorrow.

Lord I want your prayer to continue—if appropriate.

Kathy is wonderful as is everyone.

Pete had one desire that weekend, and that was to go to Crossroads on Sunday. He surprised a few people as he walked up to the Information Center, where we volunteered. They had just sent us off a week ago for brain surgery. I could almost see a strut in Pete's cautious steps. He was so proud!

My family, too, had been amazing. Our house was papered with cards and balloons and banners and flowers. My sister and niece-in-law, with their children, had decorated our home, stocked it with groceries, and made it a happy place. My nephew's daughter, Meg, age four, had presented Pete with a coffee cup painted just for him, cigar and all, with get-well wishes.

January 22, 2006—Cincinnati—Home (Pete's Journal exactly as Pete wrote it.) Challenges with word-finding start to become evident.

Let's use 2 pages.

I'm home with Kathy. We watched 2 football semifinals.

But this morning was church! Saw a few friends at the church including the Rushings and the Modeler. What a poor service though. But OK for Kathy. Then the grocery store. We did some shopping.

At home Mike stopped by shortly. Then a boater and catalogs from the marina stopped by. Craig dropped off 2 catalogs!

Kathy slowed down and we had a BIG dinner at home. Her boss called and I think he finally got my letter.

Lord, I'm watching TV. I need your help for Precents.! Miracles!

I'm forgetting names …

Church: Betty, Jerry Rushing, Steve Mercer-coop aron at church

Home: Mike, Mom & Dad, Craig Wolf

January 23, 2006—Cincinnati Home—(Pete's Journal)

At home all day. Kathy is calling her staff to talk about bonuses. She is good! Tomorrow or Wednesday we drive to Cleveland and then 100 hours! Hope I make it-with God on my side. Will walk today to dinner-Wow! At the Hill.

Thanks Lord, AND I saw the outside!! OK

Kathy and I did make a unique dinner last night at Blue Point!

I talked to all thirteen of my regional managers the day before we left for Cleveland for the second surgery. The purpose of my call was to give them their increases and bonuses for the year. It was a hard task for me. I didn't understand why it was so difficult. These were individuals whom I loved and cared for. Many had worked for me for over ten years or more. The bank had been my passion and captured my heart for the last twenty years, and I was giving them good news! Why did I have to force myself to do it? It just didn't seem important anymore.

We drove back to the Cleveland Clinic the afternoon of January 24, 2006 by ourselves. Mary Jo and Mike were going to join us later that day for dinner. Steve was flying back in from Washington DC. There was only rain; no snow. Relief.

From my prayer journal: January 24, 2006—Cleveland Clinic

I am afraid of the future, of what lies ahead. I worry about Pete's eligibility for IL-13. Will he pass the test? Will he be "good enough"? I worry about Pete's vision; I worry about the weather. And I lay my fears at your feet. Take them. I trust your plan. You will make us new. Everything in our life has changed. I don't know what life will look like on the other side of this. But I trust you will shape it in your glory. Your kingdom come. Not mine. I only get in trouble when I start worrying about what will happen to me. I've given up all the power and control of having a career. I've stripped myself of them. What will become of me? Keep me from selfishness. Self-centeredness. I turn my attention and energy to loving Pete and I know that is my calling from you-now. This is my mission to serve and comfort him. To do what matters for him. I want to do it well. With excellence. Open my eyes so I can see what he needs. Give me your guidance. Sanctify me through this process. Make me more loving. Wiser. A better representative of you. And make Pete eligible for the IL-13 treatment—please.

8

Surgery 2: The Clinical Trial Begins

"For some types of brain tumors, there is the prospect of long-term survival. This progress has been made in part through clinical trials, which are experimental studies for new treatments. Clinical trials are the best way for you to get the latest, state-of-the-art treatments. Moreover, the only way to move closer to a cure is by participation," writes Dr. Paul Zeltzer in *Brain Tumors: Leaving the Garden of Eden*. A clinical trial is "a method designed to study, scientifically, the effectiveness of a specific treatment," according to *Brain Tumors: Finding the Ark*.

For GBM brain tumor patients, clinical trials are of interest since there is no cure for brain cancer. Clinical trials are studies which, through a variety of different methods/treatments, can potentially prolong life or improve the quality of life of the patient. There are no guarantees that trials would be successful, and there were some risks with each clinical trial. Since the prognosis for Pete was so pessimistic, and his life expectancy using just the standard of care treatment was so short, we were especially open to participation in a clinical trial.

For us, the choice of which clinical trial to participate in was a matter of what the Cleveland Clinic was participating in and what Pete could be eligible for. It would have been possible to shop other national brain tumor centers to find other clinical trials to participate in, but we chose not to do so.

Usually there is a project manager for a clinical trial, and that manager is charged with making sure participants adhere to the protocol of the study."A protocol is the recipe for how the trial will be performed: eligible types of tumors, age and health of participant, drug amount and timing, type and frequency of required tests, and so forth. These variables are defined by the researchers initiating the clinical trial. It is important to know and remember that the purpose of a clinical trial is primarily the furthering of research not the recovery of any particular patient." A—*Brain Tumors: Finding the Ark*

Pete participated in the clinical trial IL-13-pe38qqr. He participated two weeks after his tumor removal as per the protocol of the study. It was January 26, 2006. The IL-13 drug was already in Phase III testing. Phase III was the last stage of research before a drug goes for approval, and is marketed to the public. If possible, it was always preferable to participate in Phase III of a clinical trial instead of Phase I or II, because so much more was known by Phase III. There were many less variables Pete had to contend with when a trial reached Phase III.

The interleukin, or IL-13, is a "naturally recurring immune system compound. As it turns out, the vast majority of glioblastoma (cells) have high levels of receptors for it, but normal brain cells have none. That means when the drug is injected directly into the brain, it seeks out the tumor cells and binds to their IL-13 receptors. The IL-13 then serves as a sort of Trojan horse that allows the deadly part of the drug PE38, a toxin produced by pseudomonas bacteria-to slip inside the tumor cell. PE38 is a nature designed killing enzyme," says a doctor involved in the trial at UC San Francisco. 'It's far more efficient at killing tumor cells than typical chemotherapy.' This quote was taken from a *Newsweek* article from December 11, 2006. The doctor involved in the trial gave great hope for IL-13, saying "This isn't a cure, but with just one treatment, we are doubling patient survival."

Pete and I both believed that his ability to have a full and high quality of life after his surgery probably had something to do with the IL-13 treatment. Others argued that the IL-13 treatment might have made him susceptible to the pneumonia that almost killed him. We could never prove the impact, because there were so many other factors that also influenced Pete's ability to live so well after surgery.

However, if given a chance to participate in another clinical trial, we would have done it again.

There is a downside in participating in a clinical trial, however. It is the realm of uncertainty that the trial puts into your future treatment. We must have asked the doctors in Cincinnati and Cleveland a hundred times, "Could the IL-13 treatment be creating this kind of scar tissue? Have other patients with IL-13 treatments had their MRIs look like this, with all this necrotic tissue?" They just didn't know. I remember one answer poignantly. I asked the project manager for the IL-13 trial, "How have other IL-13 patients fared?" desperate to get some kind of comparison twenty months after Pete's surgery. I was told that Pete was the longest-living survivor of the IL-13 trials completed at the clinic. Perhaps in the whole country. If you participated in a clinical trial, you were a pioneer. You lived with uncertainty about the impact of that trial in all your future treatments.

Pete and I drove back to Cleveland alone on January 24. I was driving this time. Pete and I went to what had become our favorite dinner place in downtown Cleveland, the Blue Point Oyster Grill. Such simple things brought us such pleasure. We had a very special and intimate dinner.

Pete and I got up early the next morning, and walked on the Cleveland Clinic campus over to the Walker Center for an appointment with the speech therapist. The Center was the furthest point on the campus from where we were staying. There were snow flurries, and a bitter wind off the lake. For the first time, Pete had trouble walking. He was dizzy. He almost fell on one of the spiral staircases. He complained of his vision being blurry, and needing to get his glasses changed. I was afraid.

The speech therapist gave us an introduction to what would be our constant challenge for the next two years. "Pete has difficulty on word retrieval due to the location of his tumor in the left temporal lobe," she said. "He'll need to use the frontal lobe for word definition, instead of what he is used to. Use sentence completion when he can't find the word in coaching him," she directed me, which would force him to use the right side of his brain. "Use sound cues," she said, and gave me an example: saying "brec" when he was searching for the word "breakfast." She gave him an assessment test with sixty items. He missed fourteen out of sixty. Looking back, I realized that was the best he would do for a long, long time.

After the speech therapist we met with Deb, the project manager for the IL-13 clinical trial. Deb started the conversation, saying Pete had some understanding problems right after the first surgery. Fear seized me. I didn't know what to expect. But then Deb kept talking, and laid out all the parameters of the IL-13 surgery for tomorrow. Dr. Barnett would insert four catheters. They would be two and a half inches long. Pete would be under anesthesia. A CAT scan would be used to verify the placement of the catheters. It would take about one hour per catheter, and two incisions per catheter. Before noon the next day the clock would start running, and the immunotoxin, IL-13 PE 38 would drip into Pete's brain for the next ninety-six hours. It all seemed so daunting to both of us.

Pete and I left that meeting with Deb, and I remember feeling ecstatic that Pete had qualified for the clinical trial. He had been good enough! I remember thanking God for getting Pete qualified for IL-13. God's faithfulness to us!

January 25, 2006—Hotel Intercontinental, Cleveland (Pete's Journal—his last entry)

4 tests today. Started with the school. I missed about 14 out of 60. To learn more; take the homework about every 2–3 days.

Finally did another physical/mental X-ray.

Tomorrow is early starts the brain holes.

Ready for Friday, Saturday, Sunday, Monday! Hope I can make it.

Kathy is wonderful!!

Steve is flying in; Mike and Mary Jo drove in from home; Michael is at home.

Saw the nurse for about 1 hour. She retested me and I'll get preliminary tomorrow.

I HOPE I make it! I would like somewhat longer to help at church.

I'm reading little, both the paper and magazines. Maybe the movies will work at the surgery.

Lord, I need your help…You set the date But I want to continue.

Lord, I believe and love you!

January 26 was the second surgery day. We reported in at 5:50 a.m. We knew the drill this time. That gave us confidence. Pete's little army was looking out for him: Mike, Mary Jo, Steve and me. We could tell from the TV screen report that Pete went into OR at 7:22 a.m. but surgery didn't even start until 11:05. The doctors spent a lot of time working with the computers to make sure everything was lined up perfectly. Something went wrong with the computer, so it took them longer than planned. Pete didn't get out of surgery into recovery until 3:45 p.m. Dr. Barnett, the surgeon, didn't call until five.

He said, "Went well. Pete's a little agitated. CAT scan was okay. I pulled two of the catheters back a little; they had initially been put in too deep. Infusion will start tomorrow."

Long day. Waiting. For some reason, I was thinking this surgery would be the easier one. I was not prepared at all for how long it was, and what was ahead for us. Somewhere, I just missed the significance and impact on Pete of this second surgery. It's always harder when you're surprised.

Pete's Carepage Entry: January 26 @ 8:44 p.m.

Just saw Pete. He recognized all of us, though he is "dopey." He is so tired from his surgery but is hungry and is already eating Jell-O and broth! You are his friend if you feed him! He is speaking most words now—no sentences—but is doing fine. Down now for the third CAT scan of the evening. He will sleep well tonight. I take comfort in knowing all of you were lifting him up all day and he made it! God is good and He once again heals through such a competent group of researchers and doctors and nurses. How grateful we are for all your support and love.

The next morning Pete could not speak much. He could say his first name, but not his last. He did not know my name. He was getting a blood transfusion, and the nurse said it took until almost four a.m. before the blood was finished. Pete wouldn't take his medicine without a lot of work from the staff. He was very confused and agitated most of the day. He couldn't say when he had surgery. He spoke a lot of nonsense stuff. Pete could not open his eyes most of the day. He did eat ice cream and some dinner. I was scared. Thank goodness for all the family around. They comforted me and kept me calm.

I got to the ICU step down unit by 6:15 a.m. the second day after surgery. Pete was awake and alert, which was a surprise. At seven

Pete was still awake, but I needed to leave his side for the nurse shift change. (I do believe a person could die during shift change, and no one would notice!) I prayed in the waiting area around the corner. By eight o'clock I came in again, and Pete had kicked off his blankets, and was trying to pull out the catheters from his head.

He kept saying, "The pumps are off. We're done! Let's go home."

I was panicked. The dressing was off Pete's head wound, and I asked the nurse who had taken the dressing off. By her silence, I figured out Pete had taken his own dressing off. I asked the nurse to call Deb Kangisser, the project manager for the IL-13 treatment. The nurse refused. I felt paralyzed. I couldn't believe she wouldn't make contact, and I didn't want to leave Pete's side. Steve had come to his dad's room by then. Steve had Deb's pager number. He paged her, and she came immediately. She told the nursing staff with some irritation that she was to be called immediately next time.

Pete seemed confused and depressed. "I want to stop. Let's go home," he said. My heart sank. He didn't want to go through with this.

Kangisser said firmly to Pete, "Do you want to stop the treatment? This is only being done for you. Do you want to stop?"

Silence. Pete was not looking up. He wasn't looking at anyone.

"You have to want this," Kangisser repeated.

Silence. Finally, Pete said he would continue.

I felt relief and dread. We were only in the first few hours, and we had ninety more hours to go.

Mike had a good idea. The big poster-size get well card that the kids had made for Pete and sent to the clinic was blank on the back. We found a black marker, and listed each hour on the poster board starting with 96, then 95, 94, 93, 92, 91, 90, 89, 88, 87, 86, and so on down to one. We posted it on the wall next to Pete's bed. As each hour passed we would, with great ceremony, put a big red X through the hour just completed. Pete could see his progress, and so could we.

Pete was tethered to a stainless steel cart that had a very sophisticated pump and monitor on it for each catheter: four catheters and four pumps and monitors. There were springs embedded in plastic that stretched from the catheter in Pete's head to the pump. The cart was on wheels so Pete could stand and move and go to the bathroom, dragging the cart behind him. But that was all the mobility he had. We

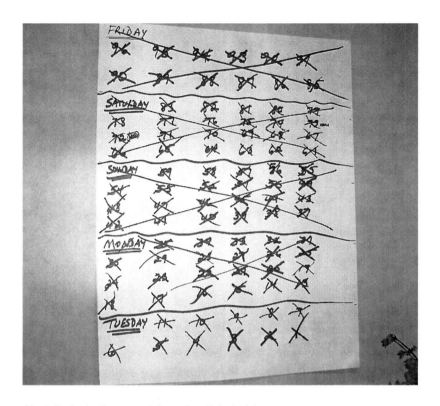

Chart displaying hour count down for clinical trial

had bought a portable DVD player and some movies. The TV was on. The hours stretched.

Pete kept saying "How long to listen to the music," which I think was a reference to the pump. He saw animals regularly. He called himself Samuel instead of Pete. I was so afraid and full of dread. The hours crawled by.

Pete's Carepage: January 28, 2006 @ 12:10 p.m.

24 hours of the 96 hours have just finished! Pete is recovering very slowly from this surgery. He still does not have his speech back and his level of understanding fades "in and out." He has been through so much. All of us think he is exhausted. Pray for his strength and endurance. He gave us all a scare today by wanting to pull his catheters out. But no harm done, he is now resting peacefully after getting cleaned up.

§ § § § §

A Pete's Carepage Response: You are an inspiration to all of us

Hi Pete. Just wanted you to know what an inspiration you are to us. You did so amazingly well after
surgery-how many people can walk around Mount Adams
and feel well enough to go to church after having
major surgery just several days prior? You got
through having the catheters inserted and if anyone
has the strength and will to get through the next 96
hours of treatment, I know you do. We are thinking
of you, and sending love and prayers your way. Your
strength, positive attitude, and faith will get you
through this. By the sheer volume of messages for
you on this site, you know all your family and
friends are there with you in spirit as well.

Tammy

§ § § § § §

Pete's Carepage: January 29, 2006 @ 11:21 a.m.

Coming up to the halfway point and Pete is more alert today. Has his glasses on and is currently watching a movie (Groundhog Day!) on his DVD player with Mike and Steve. Mike's kids, Michael J., Kevin and Ann Marie, drove up to Cleveland from Cincinnati last night to surprise us. Now—this Clinic is big! They had no idea where they were going. They "chose" the "right" parking lot out of the 6 lots that are here— and out of the 7500 patients the clinic gets every day, they walked up just as I was returning to the hospital for the next set of visiting hours. God does have a sense of humor! And they brought with them a cooler full of Graeter's ice cream—so Pete tripled his calorie intake for the day as he ate the WHOLE thing—a pint of double chocolate chip in one sitting! He was smiling. All of us had drinks at the hotel bar last night— Steve ordered us a few shots of "Jack" and I knew Pete would rather have had the "Jack." Hopefully soon.

Speech is still a problem but Pete understands everything—the docs call it a problem with "word retrieval" and they consider it a normal and temporary (we hope) side effect of the swelling in the brain from the surgery and this IL-13 treatment. His spirits are OK— pray for his strength. This is a marathon he is running!

Thanks to all for such love and wonderful messages. I told Pete, Joe (my brother in Eugene Oregon), said that he is taking you salmon fishing this Fall.

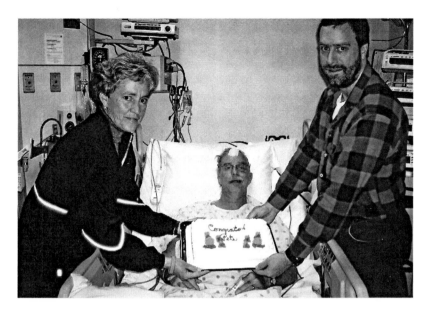

Kathy, Pete, and Steve at the clinical trial completion

This weekend we would have been at the 24 Hour Race in Daytona. Pete and I promised each other this morning that we WILL be back at the race next year. We are counting the hours as "laps" and believing in the win. You give us strength-counting on you to keep the good energy flowing this way!

PS Kevin, Mike and Ann Marie just reported another pint of Graeter's is gone!

Pete's Carepage: January 30, 2006 @ 10:42 a.m.

Steve (son) and Kevin (nephew) were able to get the soundtrack and standings from the 24 Hours Race in Daytona on their laptops so Pete and I were able to listen to the end of the race. Very exciting finish—one lap between # 1 and #2 after 24 hours! Not quite like our normal grandstand viewing but it may be the race ending that I remember most of all.

Pete's Carepage: January 31, 2006 @ 1:22 p.m.

Whooo-hoo! The IL-13 treatment is finished! That's 5 hours of surgery and 4 days (96 hours) of IL-13 infusion. The catheters were removed right on schedule as our countdown chart hit zero. So we made it. Pete successfully completed the infusion!

Next, Pete will be moved to a regular room and given a night to recover and get his sea legs back. If all goes well, we will head home tomorrow. Yes!

Pete is tired and needs some time to recover. We are so proud of him. He ran this marathon with class! Thanks to all and each of you for giving us the strength and endurance to get through this. Milestone # 2 is accomplished!

We found a place to live while in Cleveland for the next six weeks for the radiation treatments. Mike and Steve scouted it out for us. It was an apartment downtown in the Warehouse District, near lots of our favorite places. It looked out on the Cuyahoga River. There was a fitness center and a roof deck. It would be just fine, just fifteen minutes from the clinic.

My conversations with God during this second surgery had a couple of themes. I reminded God of Jeremiah 29:11, which was read at Crossroads as we started our journey to the clinic in mid-January. "I know the plans I have for you. Plans to prosper you and not to harm you, plans to give you hope and a future." I turned to God as the source of our hope. We both hoped that Pete and I would be able to do some of God's work together.

The second theme was of a healing God. I remembered the Roman centurion's story told in the Gospel of Luke. Jesus was amazed by the Centurion's faith. I wanted Jesus to be amazed by our faith, too.

I gained a perspective in those days in the clinic: Pete and I weren't the only people suffering brain tumors. Others were in much more dire straits—patients with young children, patients not able to afford treatment, patients old and dying. I realized I had made so many mistakes in my past. I had made judgments about one of our friends who had been disabled due to a stroke. I was quick to think he should have been able to do more, be less depressed. Oh, what shame I felt! I looked at Pete in that hospital bed, not able to speak, depressed himself, and unable to move or walk without help. Never again arrogance from me; judgments of others would stop.

We got home on Wednesday, February 1, knowing that we would make a return trip to Cleveland on Super Bowl Sunday, February 5. Pete needed to get fitted for his mask for radiation treatments, which were scheduled to begin February 10. So we went to Cleveland for a day, back home, then a return trip to Cleveland to move in to the apartment for at least the next six weeks on February 9.

Pete was fitted for a flexible mesh mask which would be used to hold his head in place each time he received a radiation treatment. The radiologist used Pete's MRI after surgery, lined up with the CT scan, to determine where radiation should occur. The purpose of the radiation was to kill any cancer cells in and around the tumor bed. Radiation would be every day, Monday to Friday, for about twenty to thirty minutes. Side effects would be fatigue, scalp irritation and possible increase in neurological symptoms. Receiving radiation with Temodar, a chemotherapy agent, had been shown to increase the effectiveness of radiation, and as Dr. Barnett had explained, increase Pete's life expectancy another three months. Our plan was to live in the apartment in Cleveland during these six weeks.

The trip back home after the mask-fitting was hard. Pete slept most of the way. He could not walk without assistance. His vision was blurred, and he could not focus enough to read. Dr. Barnett had said that the swelling in Pete's brain from all the treatment and fluids could be affecting his speech and be giving him double vision. It might take weeks to see improvements from those side effects. Even with those handicaps, Pete managed to get out of the car, and with Mike's help, got his Frosty at the Wendy's in Columbus, Ohio, the halfway point on the trip home. Pete weighed one hundred and fifty three pounds as we left the clinic, having lost sixteen pounds.

Pete's very fast return to normal after the actual craniotomy (surgery number one), and his subsequent slow and painful reaction to the clinical trial infusion of IL-13 (surgery number two) was a surprise. From walking the hills of our neighborhood after his brain tumor was removed to hardly being able to talk or keep his eyes open after the IL-13 surgery was a mystery. Despite all the information I had read, I was not been prepared for the side effects after either surgery. I asked lots of questions of the nurses and doctors, and listened hard for words like "this is normal" or "this is just a temporary problem." As ecstatic as I had been after Pete's first surgery, so was I now scared and worried after the second. The roller coaster of brain tumor treatment and recovery had begun!

The days at home were difficult. Pete was very tired. He napped a lot. He had difficulty walking. The right side of his foot turned on its side as he walked. He complained of dizziness. He had a tingling feeling in his right side, especially in his arm and hand. Pete said his arm always felt like it was asleep. His fine motor skills were a challenge. He couldn't hold a fork in his right hand. Dropped a lot of things. Pete was now using two hands to hold a glass. One day, he made it up the stairs and back down. He showered with my help on two of the days. He did some leg lifts with light weights, and even some speech word lists. The speech exercises forced Pete to name opposites. He got six right out of twenty.

I finally called Deb Kangisser, the project manager of the IL-13 clinical trial, and she increased Pete's dexamethasone (steroids) back up to twenty milligrams. She said the swelling in Pete's brain from the IL-13 treatment was causing Pete's symptoms, and they would disappear once the swelling went down. She said these symptoms were normal; Pete's reaction was just delayed.

Pete was very depressed. I could not really have an adult conversation with him. I felt so alone and sad myself. Pete would say, "I want to stop. I want it over. I don't want to live." My heart broke. I thought maybe I was doing something wrong. Was it the medication? Did Pete really understand what he was saying or not? My prayer was "Lord, what do I do with this?"

Pete's Carepage: February 4, 2006 @ 11:37am

We have developed a little routine here at home and it is nice to do all the normal things. Thanks for all your continued prayers and support. Cooking (me! That's a miracle!) Showering, exercising, reading and listening to the music of Pete's new satellite radio. All the Metro team at the Bank got Pete a satellite radio and brother-in-law Mike figured out how to get it working and got it registered, so Pete has 200 options of all kinds of music and talk shows. His favorite so far is classic rock-in-roll and "bluesville." Nice gift from God—you US bankers—because Pete's vision is not real good now and he can't read anything, even his "beloved" WSJ. So the radio is a great blessing!

For all of you still praying, here's the focus: on Pete's vision—that it clears up—and on his balance/motor skills. He is still having a hard time walking, and is dizzy. We keep trying to be patient (I'm about as good at that as cooking!) and hope that as his brain recovers from the swelling these obstacles will disappear. Pete is doing his "word exercises" every day that we got from the cognitive therapist, and started leg lifts with light weights so he can build up his strength. Speech is still difficult, so you can imagine his frustration! We are counting on all of you, through your prayers, to lift his spirits and strengthen his belief and hope.

I was re-listening to the Crossroads message from January 15, the day we left for the clinic for the first surgery. The theme was dreaming. Jeremiah 29:11 "I have plans for you and a future." The message was about how our dreams will be tested. Pete has his dreams and they are being tested! Your words of encouragement and outpouring of love will get him/us through these tests! Keep 'em coming and thank you! Thank you!

§ § § § §

A Pete's Carepage Response: Plans for You and A Future

I read the updates with great admiration for your focus and determination on your road to recovery. I know too well from my own experience where you are. Two years ago I lay almost dead on Interstate Rte 75, and after many surgeries I could not see like I could before and I had many dizzy and unstable spells that I could not have gotten through without the care and attention of Barbara. Every day was a new challenge, but also a new day of determination to improve and beat my "issues" and related weaknesses from the accident. Lots came from 'within,' lots came from my family and friends, and everything came from our powerful God. My eyesight has returned to where it was before, if not possibly better. The dizziness is a thing of the past. The weakness of the body when at one time a walk to the bathroom was an accomplishment, has now returned to where I can walk great distances, play golf and ski in the mountains of Colorado. What I learned in the ordeal was a word I did not know before, "patience." I know your will and determination because I have seen it before. You too will come back, because of your will AND God's will. Take a new step each day and keep your goals always in your mind. But too, remember the word "patience" and you will get there. And there are many "theres." One of the "theres" is your first trip this summer on your boat, My Destination. I look forward to being your co-captain. Tomorrow morning I again take my prayers for you up to the 35,000 foot level in route to Toronto. I know God is listening, I know God has you in his views, I know God has your road to recov-

ery well paved and that God has "plans for you and a
future."

Craig

§§§§§

On Sunday, February 5, the day we were leaving to go back to
Cleveland, Pete showered and shaved. That effort exhausted him.
Mike drove us to Cleveland. I'll never forget that dismal grey Super
Bowl Sunday in a hotel room in the Key Marriott in downtown
Cleveland, with room service pizzas, salad and a cooler of beer we
had brought with us. Pete stayed up the whole game. He was alert as
the Steelers beat the Seahawks.

On Monday, February 6, Pete weighed in at one hundred and forty
nine pounds. He had been at one hundred and sixty-even pounds before
all this began. The clinic took a blood test. Pete's platelet count was only
eighty-seven thousand. He needed to be at least a hundred thousand
before the chemotherapy agent, Temodar, could be used with the radiation. The platelet count is a blood element that promotes clotting. A low
platelet count made Pete more susceptible to bleeding. The use of Temodar with radiation had been proven to make the radiation more effective,
delaying tumor recurrence. According to the protocols for the clinical
trial, Pete had to have Temodar administered with his radiation, and both
needed to be supervised by the Cleveland Clinic. Dr. Barnett's thinking
was that the Dilantin anti-seizure medication might be causing Pete's
low platelet count. He discontinued the Dilantin, and increased Pete's
dose of Keppra. Pete was barely speaking. We used a wheelchair to get
around at the clinic, because of his dizziness and difficulty in walking.
We left to come home that Monday night, planning to return on Thursday to begin treatment and move into our apartment.

I can remember that dark drive back home in the car. Mike drove.
We spoke little. Mike had a James Taylor CD playing. Pete sat in the
passenger seat asleep, his head flopping on his chest. I sat in the back
seat with tears streaming down my face. Pete's life seemed of such
poor quality. My heart was breaking. Things seemed hopeless.

Mary Jo and Mike drove us back to Cleveland Thursday. Pete's
speech was improving. The four of us had a regular conversation at
dinner that night, even though Pete's walking was still shaky at best.
It took four of us to escort him from the elevator of the hotel across
the lobby to the restaurant. He was much too unsteady on his feet to
go out. No favorite Cleveland restaurants that night! But Pete was
talking so much better. Hope lifted its head again!

Pete's Carepage: February 12, 2006 @ 9:54 a.m.

*Sunday morning and we are all moved into our new 'home"
away from home. Our new address for the next 6 weeks is:*

Nadherny Beechem

1278 West Ninth, Apt 834

Cleveland, Ohio 44113

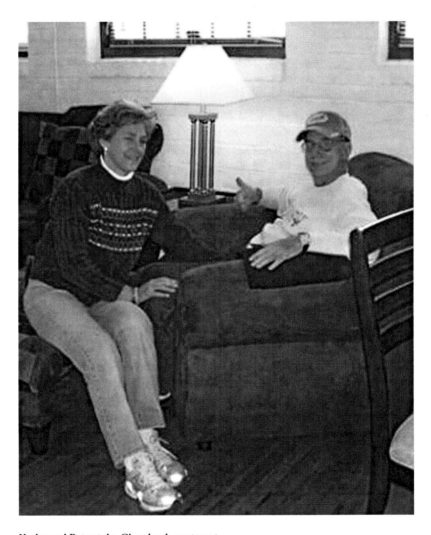

Kathy and Pete at the Cleveland apartment

It will do just fine. We even have a "river" view but, without offending my good friends from Cleveland, the Cuyahoga is NOT like the Ohio! But we do have sea gulls in the morning—I take joy in their noise as I pray. Pete is doing very well. Mary Jo and Mike were our "angels" these past days, getting us moved in and helping us get around the clinic on Friday. We would not have had a chance of doing this without them. They left late afternoon yesterday for home. Such a quiet after they left. Getting used to all the strange noises of a new place—the refrigerator and heat and coffee pot. We feel like lonely pioneers in a wilderness. But we are together and determined to have fun!

We went to a movie in a theatre at the downtown mall. With lots of effort, Pete walked all over the mall, from the parking lot to the theatre. He was very proud of himself. And I was so proud of him. Had a blast seeing "Firewall" and having dinner in the food court.

Radiation is scheduled to begin tomorrow—Monday. The docs are worried about Pete's platelet count being low, so their discussion Friday was of postponing the radiation for another week. They once again adjusted Pete's medicine, because it could be affecting the low platelet count. They really don't know what is causing this, but after we got another scan late Friday, Dr. Barnett recommended we proceed with radiation Monday if possible. So Pete and I will go to the clinic Monday and get a blood test, and if his platelet count has lifted higher (it has been trending up since the second surgery) we will start radiation. Pete's vision is clearing up some, though he still can't read much. His speech is much better! We are back to regular (and frequent) conversations now. His humor and sarcasm are back! He's walking, but still with some difficulty. As he says, "We have already seen more of the Winter Olympics that we ever wanted to or ever have before." We continue to treasure each day. Keep praying that Pete can get his "right side working better," and that his vision clears. We count on you and are strengthened by your prayers and faithful support. God keeps giving us little "treats." The latest is a wonderful gourmet grocery right in our apartment building. Pete and I toured it yesterday. The staff already knows Pete by name and is praying for him. Samura, one of the cashiers, has her whole Lebanese family engaged. Constantino's is the grocer and they have prepared foods as well as fresh produce and a deep and good wine selection (Yahoo! Great), bakery items made fresh— and lots of chocolate. How good is God?

On the same day we moved into the Cleveland apartment, we visited the doctors at the Brain Tumor Institute. They once again tested Pete's platelet count, and it was up to ninety-six thousand, still not high enough to begin the Temodar with the radiation, but close enough that the staff held a place for Pete's treatment to begin on that Monday, February 13.

There was a lot of commotion and concern about Pete's platelet count being so low. Was he bleeding? Was it the Keppra medication? They quickly scheduled another CAT scan. No bleeding, thank goodness. The oncologist changed Pete from the Keppra drug to Topamax, another anti-seizure medication, in case the Keppra was causing the low platelet count. This was now the third anti-seizure medication Pete had been on since surgery on January 16. Dr. Barnett, Pete's surgeon, was alarmed because he saw an enhancement in Pete's brain near the thalamus, which was where Pete's original tumor had been. An enhancement meant Pete's brain cells were lighting up on the scan, which in turn meant there was some activity. The tumor could be growing again. And that created in Dr. Barnett urgency around getting Pete's radiation started right away. Monday was to be the day!

Mary Jo and Mike encouraged me to think about just quitting now and heading home. Would I consider talking to Pete about ending all the treatment? "Just stop," they said. "Let Pete have as many good days as he can, and let the tumor progress as it will and deal with it as it changes."

It was a good question. It was a question that should have been asked, and would be asked, many times over the next months. The medical system usually never asks that question. Their job is to do whatever is necessary to keep Pete alive. The question of the quality of that life really rests with the patient and the caregiver. For now, I couldn't even consider stopping. It felt like giving up to me. I wanted Pete to keep fighting as long as he possibly could. I guess his fight was my source of hope. I never brought the question up to Pete.

Pete and I reported into the huge reception area of Building R/20 at the Brain Tumor Institute on Monday morning. We had the routine down: register at one window, then head to another window for blood tests. Afterward, we sat in the waiting area. Deb, the project manager from the IL-13 Clinical trial, came out to greet us. She told us there was no way we could start the Temodar chemo with the radiation today. Pete's platelet count had dropped back to eighty-seven thousand from ninety-six thousand on Friday, and the threshold was one hundred thousand. We would have to wait another week to start radiation, if Pete's platelet count would rebound enough to begin with the Temodar. However, the only reason to wait to start radiation was because of the parameters of the clinical trial. The study required "radiation with Temodar post IL-13 infusion." I could feel the tension building within me.

Finally, Dr. Barnett weighed in: "Forget the study. Pete needs to get radiation started now! He can add Temodar to his treatment at a later date any time."

The consequence of that recommendation was that Pete would not complete the clinical trial, since he was not going to be able to meet the strict parameters. Dr. Barnett was recommending what Pete needed, not what the study required. I felt so appreciative of Dr. Barnett! We quickly all concluded that we might as well go home and get Pete's radiation done in Cincinnati, since the clinic would no longer need to supervise. "Wanna go home?" I asked Pete.

He broke into the biggest smile! I called Mary Jo and Mike in Cincinnati from the reception area in R/20 while Deb waited. Mary Jo and Mike dropped everything, got in their car and started the four-hour trip back to Cleveland to pick us up and move us out of the apartment. Deb assured me that the clinic would still be available to us even though Pete was no longer in the clinical trial.

As Deb said, "Pete got the benefit of the IL-13 treatment; the study is now more hassle than it's worth."

How thankful I was for the generosity of the Cleveland Clinic staff. I valued their decision to do the right thing for Pete, and not base their care decisions on their impact to their research results. By that same evening Pete and I were safely home, thanks once again to our angels Mary Jo and Mike who, in a span of twelve hours, drove four hours to pick us up, moved all of our belongings and groceries out of the apartment, and drove with us another four hours back home to Cincinnati.

From my prayer journal: Valentine's Day, 2006

> *We are home. I give you thanks for getting us home and back to our sources of support. Pete is comfortable here at his home. So am I. Thank you for safe travels, and for the angels you send in Mary Jo and Mike. Help me not be afraid. No Valentine's Day cards this year, nor dinners out, but I am thankful to have my Valentine. Thank you for each day we have. I cannot see the way, but I know you are leading us. Pete needs your protection. Protect us both under your wing.*

9

The Darkest Days

Pete was in a fog. He wouldn't shower or shave. Pete slept a good part of every day. His vision got worse. He was confused. Mobility was a problem. As I look back, the fog was probably created by the two anti-seizure medicines Pete was on. The doctors couldn't stop the Keppra right away, but started the Topamax. So we had a tapering schedule to follow for the Keppra, and an increasing dosage for the Topamax. The tapering schedule was about four weeks. Pete's blood pressure was low for him, in the 117/72 range.

Pete didn't want to take any medicine. Each time his medicine was scheduled, it was a fight between Pete and me. I felt out of control. I felt angry because he was being so stubborn. I was afraid of failing as a caregiver if I couldn't get him to take his pills. Mary Jo had researched the Topamax drug, and one of the side effects was depression. She wanted me to stop giving Pete the Topamax. I was afraid to do that without a doctor's order. The possibility of seizures terrified me. I would have suggested it to a doctor, but I couldn't get Pete into see a doctor. Since we were now no longer under the care of the clinic, the only Cincinnati doctor we had was a surgeon, Dr. Warnick. But Pete didn't need a surgeon. He needed what I soon learned to call "a neuro-oncologist." Dr. Warnick recommended Dr. Albright. We couldn't get anyone from Albright's office to return my calls. I was panicking. Pete was miserable, and I had no one that could help him.

We did make it in to see a radiologist. Dr. Barnett had given me a healthy sense of urgency around getting Pete's radiation started right away. The radiologist was kind to us, but we had to have another initial visit where we told Pete's story once again. *How many times have we done this?* I thought in frustration and impatience.

Now Pete had a new set of doctors and new set of staff. The radiologist told us that Pete would need thirty-three days of radiation treatment. The biggest side effect would be tiredness, and possibly some hair loss. It would be unusual for him to experience nausea or headaches. It was not unusual if he experienced some change in taste, since his saliva glands were right in line with the area to receive radiation. He also said Pete might feel some ear pressure and fluid buildup for the same reason. The radiologist needed to do his own mask for Pete, so now Pete had to go through the process again of getting another mask done here. Another MRI. Another CAT scan. More blood tests.

I called the Cleveland Clinic. In desperation, I begged them to help Pete. They adjusted down the Keppra a little, and decreased the steroids some. My panic continued. The nurse at the clinic knew Dr. Albright and Dr. Albright's physician assistant. She said she would help get their attention on Pete.

Jerry Deese, Pete's best friend from Florida, came in. He provided a little lift to Pete's spirits. He went with us for Pete's MRI, and to the hospital for more blood tests. Jerry got Pete out of the house for the first time (other than to a hospital) since he returned from the clinic. It was always our tradition to take Jerry to his favorite Cincinnati ribs place when he visited. So with a shaky walk, Jerry and I on each side of him, Pete walked into the best ribs place in the country! He was determined not to disappoint Jerry.

We finally got a call back from Dr. Albright's office, but Pete's appointment was a week away. Albright's nurse told me that it was normal for Pete to be so knocked out with the combined medicines. "Hang in there," she said when I asked her about dropping the Topamax. Dr. Albright was in agreement with the Cleveland Clinic's strategy to get Pete off of Keppra and on to Topamax. He was convinced that the Keppra was keeping Pete's platelet count depressed. "It just takes time," she said to me.

On the way home from the airport, having dropped Jerry off, Pete spoke up angrily. "This is it," he said. "End it all."

"No, I won't end it all. I won't stop everything," I said. "Are you angry?"

"Yes," he said. "Jerry doesn't have this disease. I do. Jerry keeps getting to do all the good stuff. I don't."

I didn't know what to do with his anger. It was the first time since his diagnosis that I heard him express it. I told him I could understand why he felt that way. I was scared.

Pete became obsessed with the idea that I needed to return to work. "When are you returning to the bank?" he would ask me. "Don't you have a business trip you need to go on?" He would repeat this question over and over, many times during each day.

"Call Richard," he would say. "Tell him you are ready to go back. Richard promised me he would look after you, and that you could go back any time you want."

I kept telling Pete I felt no need to go back to work. I didn't want to be anywhere but with him. The bank would be just fine without me. Pete would then plead and beg me to end it all. I was full of despair.

Radiation finally began on February 22, 2006. It had been eight days since we had left the clinic. Pete could have been eight days further in his treatment if we hadn't come home. But home was the right decision. We both felt peaceful about that. I was just frustrated it took so long to get radiation started here. Dr. Barnett's warning that the tumor could be growing again replayed in my mind, and filled me with urgency and fear.

Pete's steroid dosage was being tapered down. The Keppra was being tapered down. Pete was still pretty knocked out. He had developed a cough, and I could hear congestion in his lungs. He became confused about time of day, whether it was a.m. or p.m. He was very difficult to physically move. He couldn't sit up from a lying position without help. Steps were painfully difficult. I had counted sixteen stairs to get from our bedroom up to the living area. Eight steps to get from the bedroom to the car. I had to dress Pete completely one day, and I don't know if he couldn't dress himself or wouldn't dress himself because he was so depressed. Pete cried that morning when I woke him up. He pleaded and begged me to stop.

Bill came to our house that day to do Healing Touch on Pete, as he had been doing since we got home from the clinic. As soon as he walked through our front door and into our living room, Bill felt a surge of energy hit him. The door was about twenty feet from where Pete sat in his favorite chair.

Bill stopped dead in his tracks. "The archangels are here. I felt the intense energy all the way out here," Bill said, his hands and arms reaching out, and touching the air like he was holding a big room-size bubble.

"Who is here?" I asked.

"Well, let's see," Bill said with a laugh in his eyes. "We have the company of Michael, Gabriel and Uriel. All archangels coming to be with you, Pete," Bill said in a hushed voice. "God sure loves you, Pete."

I was dumbstruck in amazement. All I could do was give thanks. It was a sacred moment. A little spark of hope rekindled inside me. I thanked God for sending His messages through Bill and Nan. I trusted Bill, and would try to find a way to follow whatever Bill directed me to do. I believed God was healing Pete through Bill.

Richard, my boss at the bank, called shortly thereafter. I told him about how Pete was obsessing about me going back to work. I complained that I couldn't get him to stop. Richard simply said, "Tell him you have decided that you are going back. Stop fighting him."

Duh! Richard was right. I did as he suggested. I told Pete I'd be going back to work, and we would talk about a date later on. That ended Pete's pleading. Pete never brought up my returning to work again. God does send angels.

I read C.S. Lewis' *Mere Christianity* during this difficult time. It was the second time I read it, but this time I was very moved. I began to see more of my own evil. The concept of moral law made new sense to me. "Christianity has nothing to say to people who do not know they have done anything to repent of and who do not feel that they need any forgiveness. It is after you have realized that there is a Moral Law, and a Power behind that law, and that you have broken that law and put yourself wrong with that Power—it is after all this, and not a moment sooner, that Christianity begins to talk."

I saw that I had spent most of my twenties writing my own rules. I had made my own laws. I thought of myself as my own god. I had rebelled against society's mores, and the commands of Christianity. My arrogance justified my rebellion. I was special and above others. The rules didn't apply to me.

The sexual promiscuity of my twenties was my power play, seducing different partners too numerous to count. I was twenty-nine years old when I met Pete. He was thirty-five years old, married and with two sons. I was still operating in the mode of wanting what I wanted, and paying no real regard to his family, his current wife and the pain, hurt and disruption I caused. It never occurred to me. That realization made me feel shame. Still does.

Pete clearly saved my life from a spiral that was spinning in the wrong direction. Pete called me to something higher. He taught me about commitment, because he expected it. Out of love for him and faithfulness to him, I was never sexually promiscuous again. God did indeed bring good out of an evil situation. How thankful I was for Pete! I could care for him for many years and never repay the debt I owed him. He literally saved my life.

Though no longer promiscuous, my pride and arrogance were still very alive within me. They just showed up in new forms of expression. Through caring for Pete, I was becoming humbler, a much gentler and more patient person. I could see how I was changing while I was changing. I began to feel more compassion for others, through my compassion for Pete. This transformation would be the start of a lifelong journey for me.

Pete's Carepage: February 21, 2006 @ 3:00 p.m.

We have been blessed by so many of you in helping us through "slogging" times. Thanks for all your messages and good wishes and powerful prayers. We are still struggling, but a little good news is helping us clear the way. Pete's radiation has started and will continue for the next six weeks every day, except we get a break on the weekends. Pray for his strength to endure these. Mary Jo (sister) also helped rattle some cages of our docs—the Cleve Clinic and the Cincinnati doc (thank goodness for RNs talking to other RNs) and got the schedule escalated for getting Pete off the dual medication which has Pete so "zonked." So instead of a whole week more of this, it is hopeful we might have him down to one anti-seizure medicine by Thursday or Friday. Yeah! And finally, for all your praying for his healing, we are lucky enough to have a good friend, Bill Dillon, who is certified in Christian Healing Touch. Bill did healing touch with Pete today and reports that Pete had a real spiritual surge—archangels and all filling him and fighting for him. Bill has committed to help Pete through radiation by doing healing touch each day after radiation, to help cleanse his body from the bad effects of the radiation in the rest of his body. This may help in easing the fatigue of the treatments. God is good. He continues to send his messengers in all kinds of forms. We received a prayer quilt yesterday from the So California, Arizona and Nevada US Bank training team. Each knot of the quilt represents a prayer said for Pete. How loving is that!

That same day, Pete got a letter from the White House. Pete and I both smiled. Steve was at work. The White House sent it to our home. Steve posted it on his dad's Carepage. Pete smiled again. Steve was proud. Here's the letter to Pete from George W Bush.

Dear Pete:

Laura and I want to send you a letter of encouragement. You are in our thoughts and prayers.

We hope the support of your family and friends is of great comfort to you during this difficult time. Your strength and determination demonstrate the American spirit. May God bless you and your family.

Sincerely,

George W. Bush

It was February 23, 2006, and Pete's second radiation treatment was complete. We finally had our first visit to the neuro-oncologist, Dr. Albright. It had been ten days since we came home from Cleveland. Pete weighed in at one hundred and forty-eight pounds. He had now lost almost twenty pounds, and his blood pressure was 94/62.

Mary Jo went with us to the doctor. This started a habit we would follow over the next two years. Mary Jo, Mike or Paula, my sister-in-law who was also a registered nurse, would go with us to doctor visits. They would have our medical journal and take notes, which allowed Pete and me to focus totally on what the doctor was saying. Many times we would prepare questions with them before the visit, and trade notes while in the waiting room. So helpful!

I could tell immediately that Dr Albright was aggressive. He blurted out his assessment of Pete in rapid fire. "We are going after this thing!" he said. "We will fight for life, but the race is already lost. We can try to stop the tumor from growing. It looks like it is moving toward the back of your brain, toward the brain-stem, Pete, which is a bad place. We will try some aggressive therapies: an immunotherapy called Avastin, as a last run. We'll slow the growth through the radiation and chemotherapy. And then in a few weeks, I'll be able to tell if the tumor growth has slowed down and know the time frame."

He took a breath. "Avastin is sometimes hard to get approved by insurance," he said. "It is very expensive."

"That is not a problem," I said. "I'll make a call."

And I did. I called Richard while we were still in the doctor's office. He was in California, but happened to be traveling with the head of human resources for the bank. He handed the phone to her.

She told me, "The bank is self-insured. The insurance company only acts as an administrator of our insurance plan. You should not worry. The bank would approve payment for any treatment that Pete needs."

What relief that gave me. I felt a little pride in my company, as I walked in and told Dr. Albright that the Avastin would not be a problem. It had taken me all of about fifteen minutes to get an answer!

We were at the doctor's office for hours. Dr. Albright immediately started treating Pete. He started depakote intravenously, another anti-seizure medicine that would relieve the Keppra/Topamax double-whammy effects. He also gave Pete medication for his high blood sugar. Pete sat in a wheelchair during the whole visit, and looked pretty bad.

Albright said Pete had a lot of things out of balance. Later, he told me that he told his friends at the Cleveland Clinic they had sent Pete home in pretty bad shape! His platelet count had now dropped to fifty thousand. His blood sugar was high—over four hundred (normal is 80–110). Pete had pneumonia, and the swelling in his ankle signaled a possible blood clot. Dr. Albright embraced it all, and the lion in this doctor roared. Dr. Albright was in Pete's corner, and the fight was on against this tumor. I liked him immediately, as did Pete. I was also terrified.

Mary Jo cornered the doctor and his assistant, Nancy, while Pete was getting treated. She told them about Pete's depression, which we had mentioned days earlier on the phone, and asked the doctor if they thought the end was near. Should we stop the drugs and everything now, and get hospice in and just keep Pete comfortable? Nancy told Mary Jo not to worry. When that was the appropriate step we would know, and Nancy and the doctor would help us know when that time was. But not now.

Michael came in from Florida for a visit the day before our doctor's visit. Even Pete's sick eyes lit up, so happy to see him! Michael decided to make a dinner of all dinners for his dad, so Michael didn't join us at the doctor's office. He stayed home and cooked.

Michael is a great chef. He had worked in the restaurant business since high school. He bought the choicest ingredients he could find in Cincinnati: filet mignon and mashed potatoes made with cream. Fresh asparagus. Good wine. Michael just poured love into that meal!

When we got home from the doctor's, Pete rested as Michael finished cooking. Pete got himself to the table, and the three of us sat down for the feast. Pete tried so hard to stay awake and eat, but he couldn't. His head nodded. He could only manage a few bites. Dinner was over. My heart broke for Michael and for Pete. I remember cleaning up the kitchen in the silence and the coming darkness. It was one of my loneliest moments.

The next day Pete stayed in bed, and I took food downstairs to the bedroom and fed him. I began recording what he ate: three ounces of yogurt, orange juice, four ounces of milk. I cancelled the Doppler exam that would determine if Pete had blood clots, because I could not get Pete up and to the hospital by his appointment time. Lunch was four to five shrimp that Michael had prepared as an hors d'oeuvre the night before. Michael helped me feed his dad. He was so tender and loving with his father. Dinner was a small bowl of mashed potatoes, and a few bites of meatloaf. One spoon of Jell-O. Sips of milk.

Michael helped me get his dad dressed, up the eight stairs to the garage, and into the car so we could get Pete to his radiation treatment. We did it. Felt like a huge accomplishment. Pete was so weak. He was able to walk back down the stairs to our bedroom, but with some difficulty. His breathing was very labored. He tired so easily. Going to the bathroom left him exhausted. I didn't know what was wrong. I was scared. I was checking his temperature constantly, but he had no fever. The cough worsened.

Michael left to return home early Saturday. Nan and Bill came to our home for Pete's daily healing touch treatment. Pete was in bed downstairs. Looks of worry were exchanged between me and Nan and Bill. In the month now that Pete had been receiving Healing Touch from Bill, this was the first time Pete was in bed without the strength to get up the stairs to his favorite chair.

From my prayer journal: February 24, 2006

Make me not afraid, I prayed. I cannot see the way you are leading us, protect us under your wing.

I ask for you to drive out Pete's demons. His sense of despair. Loss. Depression. You are more powerful than drugs. You are more powerful than cancer cells. You can heal him physically and spiritually. Give Pete your life. Let him rejoice in you.

How much longer, Lord? No improvement. How difficult for Pete and me! Give us some hope. Some sign of change for the better today. Please. My plea. Hear me. I'm knocking.

Should I try to help Pete deal with his own death? Walk by him. I don't know how to do this. Should I focus on dealing with my own death and sharing that with him? How terrifying!

I surrender to you as I surrender my life to Pete's care.

The doc says we have already lost the race. You are more powerful than all the docs. You are more powerful than all medicine. What do you say? Only you make the race done. If this is your will-so be it. I submit and surrender to you. I'll stop asking for what I want: To have more life with Pete. I give up what I want because I trust you and I know you are good and you are better than I can ever imagine. But like the widow and the heartless judge-you told us to keep praying. Be persistent. Never quit. Keep asking. All the people supporting us keep asking for us, too. May your healing grace find a home in Pete. Give him healing in his body. Stop the growth of this tumor. Kill all the cancer cells. Give him healing of his spirit. Give him your comfort. Peace. Let him rest in you.

10

Though I Walk Through the Valley of Death (Psalm 23)

Pete's Carepage: February 25, 2006 @ 4:40 p.m.

Join me in calling on all the archangels; we need a few spirit warriors with their swords brandished about now.

Mary Jo and Mike stayed with Pete so I could go to the Crossroads' Saturday night service. When I came home, Pete was in bed propped up with pillows. I told him about the service message of God's love and God as the source of life. He listened intently, not able to say a word. As I talked, tears streamed down my face. I told him of God's love, and my love for him. The smile on Pete's face as he listened about the message and the music lit up the whole room!

The next morning Pete was very labored in his breathing. Mary Jo and Mike came back over early in the morning to help me assess how Pete was doing. The visiting nurse came to our home that day. He told me Pete needed to go to the emergency room. The nurse confirmed that Pete was dehydrated, and had a low oxygen level. I asked him, if we didn't do the emergency room, what my other option was. He told me he didn't think I could continue to care for him in the condition Pete was in. If I didn't want to go to the hospital's emergency room, the nurse would call hospice in, and try to keep Pete comfortable.

I called Dr Albright. It was Sunday morning, but he called right back. "I am not surprised that Pete needs to go to the hospital. I almost admitted him myself when I saw him on Thursday," he said. "I'll call the emergency room so they will have orders when you arrive. And call 911; don't take him in on your own or you will be stuck waiting all day." Dr. Albright continued: "You can either take Pete to Good Samaritan Hospital, and I'll be able to care for him, or you can take him to University Hospital where he can get radiation, but I don't have hospital rights to University." He paused, waiting for my answer.

What an awful set of choices, I thought. We could go to University Hospital where Dr. Brennaman could continue Pete's radiation, but Pete couldn't have Dr. Albright caring for him. We'd have the doctor who was on call for neurology. Or we could go to Good Samaritan Hospital and have Dr. Albright, but Dr. Brennaman didn't do radiation at Good Samaritan. Either continue radiation for Pete—or have Dr. Albright. It appeared Pete couldn't have both.

"We want you." I said. "Make it Good Sam."

Pete was in the emergency room until five p.m., and then moved to the Intensive Care Unit. An IV was set up to increase Pete's fluids, and Pete began receiving oxygen right away. Pete's oxygen level popped right back up. Pneumonia was present. Strong antibiotics were ordered. Pete's platelet count had dropped to thirty-two thousand. Pete ate very little food. I went home for the evening.

That night Pete refused to take his anti-seizure pill and the nurse panicked. The nurse tried to get an IV order, but couldn't get a doctor to respond. She didn't call me. In her panic, she got a resident doctor on call to order the drug Haldol to calm Pete down, so he'd take his medicine. Giving Pete Haldol because he was refusing to take his medicine was like fixing a crack in your windshield by getting your front end replaced. Pete was zonked out. It would be days before he would get alert again. I was angry.

Dr. Albright came in and was upset about the nurses' decision from the night before. He apologized to me. I felt so responsible and mad at myself. I should have made sure Pete had all his medicine before I left to go home. I learned that I needed to protect Pete from well-meaning, but not so confident or competent nursing staff. I gave strict instructions to call me next time they had trouble getting Pete to take his medicine. I watched while they wrote that instruction in his chart. And they would call me occasionally from then on. I would try to get Pete to take all his medicine before I would leave the hospital for the night. But sometimes, about eleven at night, the phone would ring. It would be the night shift nurse.

"I can't get Pete to take his medicine," she'd say.

I'd ask for the phone while the nurse stayed near Pete. "It's all right to take your medicine, Pete. You need to, Honey. The shot is okay. The pill is okay. It's okay to take them from Tina or Penny or Michelle," I'd say.

And that would be that. He'd take the medicine, and it would be over. The nurses, who were young and lacked confidence, were the ones who usually called me. When a veteran nurse had Pete, there would never be a problem. I learned to case out the night shift nurse before I left for the evening, so I could anticipate what kind of night we were going to have. What a difference an individual makes! Thank goodness we had more night shift nurses that were experienced, caring, confident and able to handle Pete, than un-caring or inexperienced ones.

Sitting in a hospital for as many days as I had done since the first of this year gave me a pinhole look into the medical system. I had observed two hospitals at work; a half-dozen doctors, and a multitude of nurses and technicians. It can best be described as a loose system of specialties.

For example, the brain tumor staff at the Cleveland Clinic recommended that we visit Pete's primary care doctor, because they were neurologists and couldn't treat things like blood pressure. This example got repeated multiple times with each side effect, whether that was blood pressure, high blood sugar or diarrhea. Each medical team was specialized. The neurologists treated just Pete's brain tumor, even though the medicine they prescribed for treatment of the tumor might have been causing other side effects.

I soon figured out that as Pete's caregiver, one of my roles was to become Pete's advocate, and coordinate the specialists. Doctors were like the blind men feeling the elephant in the well-known story. Each blind man thought the elephant looked different, depending on their touching his trunk or his feet or his tail. They sincerely and competently thought their perspective was the right one, and usually it was. The trouble was, just like the blind men, their description of their part of the elephant was accurate, but all the described parts still didn't describe the whole. No one had the job to touch the whole elephant. Whether I wanted to or not, if Pete was going to be cared for well, I needed to become the person who touched the whole elephant. I became the advocate for Pete, and made sure the specialists talked to each other and coordinated treatment.

If the neurologist wouldn't treat Pete's blood pressure, Pete's primary care doctor became very important to us. I needed to make sure he was current on Pete's condition, so he could step in and treat whatever any given specialist wouldn't. I learned an important lesson in the case of Pete's blood pressure. We had visited Dr. Smith, Pete's primary care doctor, before Pete was hospitalized for pneumonia. His blood pressure was below one hundred. Yikes! All the dizziness and balance issues Pete had been experiencing wasn't from his brain swelling due to tumor surgery, but it was from his blood pressure medicine. I felt so bad that I hadn't figured that out earlier! As Pete had lost weight, he didn't need the same dosage of blood pressure medicine he had been on before he got sick. It had never occurred to me or to any of his doctors. We could have given him such relief, if identified earlier.

This lesson for me was about taking all of Pete's symptoms seriously. And push, push, push for treatment until the symptom was alleviated, or we understood it couldn't be fixed. I learned not to assume a doctor was right because he was an expert. He would see the problem from only one perspective. I needed to ask all the dumb and obvious questions. I learned how to "look like a lamb and be sly like a fox."

That blood pressure lesson was now being put to the test in the hospital where Pete was being treated for pneumonia. Dr. Albright, Pete's neuro-oncologist, got Pete admitted to the hospital. But he only treated Pete's brain tumor. He got hospitalists to care for everything else. I only figured this out after I looked to Dr. Albright to treat Pete's high blood sugar, which was being caused by the steroids Dr. Albright had prescribed, and I got an irritated response: "Go to your primary care doc for that."

One of the hospitalists explained to me that primary care doctors couldn't afford to make hospital rounds, because they needed to see about thirty patients a day to make a living, based on the amount of their insurance reimbursements. They couldn't do that and still make hospital rounds. So when Pete really needed his primary care doctor the most, his primary care doctor didn't see him. Instead, hospital doctors did the primary care doctors job.

Pete had a hospitalist for his primary care doctor while in the hospital, and that is why Dr. Albright wanted us at Good Samaritan. He knew the hospitalists there, and had confidence in them. The hospital doctor called in a lung doctor for Pete's pneumonia, and a heart doctor got called in because the fluid showing up in Pete's chest x-ray could be a heart problem, not just a lung problem. Dr. Albright, doing us a favor, would take charge of Pete's blood count issues so we didn't need some other specialist doctor called in for that. So Pete had Dr. Albright, a neuro-oncologist, a hospitalist, a lung doctor and a heart specialist. That's how I figured out that my job was to be Pete's advocate and make sure there was coordination among all the specialists and the hospitalists. Seemed like a weird system to me. Wondered what happened to all the people in the hospital who didn't have a me?

While Pete was in the hospital, my relationship with God changed. I was so afraid. I cried out to God. He answered me. My trust in him deepened. I expressed this deeper level of trust by a phrase, "You are the path." This phrase came from Max Lucado's book *Traveling Light,* in the chapter on hopelessness.

Max told us to imagine ourselves in a jungle, lost and alone. I had gotten lost in my early twenties in the Daniel Boone National Park in Kentucky, so it was easy for me to imagine being really lost. I had gotten separated from friends, and didn't know how to get back. I had lost all sense of direction. It had been several hours, and darkness was descending. I realized I had no food or water or tools, and I got scared. Really scared. When Max told me to imagine being lost in a jungle, I easily imagined that feeling.

Then Max asked us to just as vividly imagine getting rescued. What would that be like? What would you want? "A person, obviously. Not just an equally confused and lost person, but rather a person who knew the way out. And from this person you needed encouragement—we'll get you out. But not just encouragement but direction, 'I know how.'"

As Max says, "If you only have a person but no renewed vision, all you have is company. If he has a vision but no direction, you have a dreamer for company. But if you have a person with direction—who can take you from this place to the right place—then, you have someone who can restore your hope… Note: You haven't left the jungle. The trees still eclipse the sky and the thorns still cut the skin. Animals lurk and rodents scurry. The jungle is still a jungle. It hasn't changed, but you have. The guide before you has a machete and is hacking away the tall weeds and underbrush. You, the traveler wearied and hot, ask in frustration, 'Where are we? Do you know where you are taking me? Where is the path?' The seasoned guide stops and looks back at you and replies, 'I am the path.'" (From *Traveling Light)*

What I learned from this story was that God was the path out of the jungle for Pete and me. We were in a jungle—an ugly, scary, not very friendly jungle beset by lots of demons and horrible sounds. There wasn't any guidebook that I could use to figure out how to get Pete and me out of this jungle. I couldn't lead us out. Pete couldn't lead us out. There were no directions. Only a person. That person was Jesus. And he had vision and purpose that would lead us out.

So whenever I got afraid, I would remind myself, "You are the path." Not that you'd make a path for me and Pete to follow. But **You** are the path. "Keep my eyes fixed on you," I'd tell myself. My fears would leave. I'd feel trust and safety. My love for Pete would overflow. I learned then that fear and love can't exist at the same time. I either felt fear or felt love. If I focused on loving Pete, the fear would disappear. And I could focus on loving Pete, because I trusted in God to be the path.

While Pete was in ICU, death hovered over him. Many of my family thought this was the end. Pete was barely responsive. Pete's platelet count dropped to twenty-one thousand. Dr. Albright said he'd have to give Pete a platelet transfusion. He also needed a feeding tube.

"Nutrition is baseline," Dr. Albright said. "Any calorie Pete is taking in is getting eaten up by fighting the pneumonia, and from the steroid effect. Pete's body can't heal without nutrition. The feeding tube will give him what he needs. Pete also needs a port installed in his shoulder for access, since his veins are very fragile from the steroids. Pete is looking at a long hospital stay."

I dreaded the thought of Pete on a feeding tube. It felt horrible. And I wasn't sure he would accept the tube. Everything was moving in the wrong direction. There was one piece of good news—and it was welcome good news! The lung doctor said that Pete's body was responding to the antibiotics, and that the pneumonia was getting better. Later he told me that being on steroids actually helped Pete fight the pneumonia. Go figure!

The nurse and I had gotten the feeding tube down Pete while he was still too groggy to fight us, but by the next morning he was sitting up on the side of the bed trying to get to the bathroom. The feeding tube was out. He stood up and got into a chair. I smiled at him. He was showing his defiance! He was off oxygen.

His platelet count had gone up to sixty thousand after the transfusion. That allowed the doctors to put a PICC line into Pete's arm without his bleeding to death. A PICC line was a long tube inserted in Pete's arm. It became a form of intravenous access that was used over and over again. It allowed blood to be drawn or medicines to be injected without sticking a new needle into his veins each time.

A swallowing evaluation was done. The doctors were searching for the cause of Pete's pneumonia, and thought perhaps he was having trouble swallowing due to the brain tumor. They thought he might have experienced silent aspiration, which meant food would have gotten down into his lungs instead of his stomach, and caused the pneumonia. Pete passed the test. No swallowing problems. I sighed in relief. Another answered prayer.

As good as news was one day, bad news would follow the next. A roller-coaster was a pretty good description of what Pete's illness was like. Pete's platelet and hemoglobin blood counts dropped significantly. Was Pete bleeding from somewhere internally? If so, where? Or was the drop in blood counts just from the radiation starting again? The doctors asked the question with some urgency.

Pete became incontinent. He was back on oxygen. I got a call at home around 10:45 one night from a nurse who panicked about Pete not taking his medicine. I talked to Pete on the phone and got him calmed down, and he took his medicine. She mentioned to me that she had given Pete a dose of Lasix, because she was worried about fluid around his heart. She thought she heard fluid when she listened to his chest. I lay back down in bed, thinking the immediate crisis was over. Then I thought about what she had just said. "Lasix," I said out loud. "Oh my gosh! Poor Pete!"

I called the nurse back. "Did you say you gave him Lasix? It's 11:30 at night, and you gave him Lasix? He'll need to get up and go to the bathroom all night. He can barely walk! Why did you do that? His heart is fine!" I said with some intensity.

All I got was a mumbled answer. I jumped out of bed, pulled on some clothes and drove like lightning to the hospital. I walked into Pete's room.

He opened his eyes, "Oh, you came just in time!" he said with relief in his eyes.

I got the urinal to him and he filled it with over 500 cc's of urine. I slept next to him the remainder of the night. He had to urinate again at 12:30 and 1:30 and 3:30 a.m. All because of a nurse named Audrey. And my heart broke again.

Pete's Carepage: March 2, 2006 @ 9:15 p.m.

*Your prayers are working. God is listening and has been busy!
Pete has had two good days. Pete responded to the antibiotics for the
pneumonia and, although not off oxygen yet, needs less and less. The
docs think he has turned the corner on the pneumonia. Yeah! He is
out of intensive care and is on a "heart monitoring" floor so the nursing staff is more available. He had some heart "scares" and some
blood infection "scares" but all of these turned out not to be problems! The latest victory won today was passing the "swallowing" X-
ray test showing that he could eat for the first time in forty-eight
hours. Our nephew Kevin and his wife Ann Marie made some homemade manicotti for dinner for us, so we will always remember the
wonder of those first bites! Yum! And I don't think a Pepsi ever tasted
so good! Pete remains very weak, but he is talking and is much more
alert. He even got mad at me tonight, so he is feeling better! Praise
God for the strangest things. Next task is to build his strength, which
is all about nutrition and some therapy that can now begin. Radiation
treatments have begun again, which is a minor miracle in itself. Since
he had prepared for radiation at a different location, it was question-
able if radiation could continue at Good Samaritan hospital, and our
fear was that these treatments would be delayed. Somehow with the
radiologist working with Dr A, a way to get it done at Good Sam was
found! I still don't know how that was accomplished. Bill continues to
come every day and do healing touch with Pete-after each radiation
treatment. Such faithfulness. We are blessed.*

*Pray now for the return of Pete's strength and that he will eat
enough to get his strength back. He will remain in the hospital for a
while until he builds that back. Pray also for his spirit-the hard work
is just beginning here and he will have to have strong drive and hope
to make all the therapies—physical, cognitive, and occupational—
effective.*

*As ever—even in the dark moments—I feel and Pete feels the lift
from your prayers and love and support. Thank you a million times.*

For the rest of the week in the hospital, we got into a routine. I
would be at the hospital by eight a.m. and stay until about nine p.m.
We marked the days with little successes like getting into the chair or
taking a shower! The male nurse, Mike, was so kind to Pete, and
shaved him one evening. Kind nurses are God's angels.

Family members gave me periodic mornings off. One of them
would stay with Pete so I could stay at home a little later and exercise.

SO FAR, SO GOOD

Such gifts meant so much to me. We would have five to six visitors a day. Pete continued to get platelet transfusions since his platelet count dropped back to twenty-one thousand. Pete would sit in the chair in his room and I would take him for rides down the hospital corridor, because the chair had wheels. At the end of one of the corridors was a big picture window. He loved to sit in the sun. He told me on one of those chair trips, with the sun shining in his face and his eyes closed, "I want to work at growing the church."

"Great," I said.

Here was a man who had just gotten out of intensive care, and he's telling me in one of his first full sentences that he wanted to grow the church? Pete had not ever expressed this before. I wondered. I remembered that Pete was always so excited when Crossroads would report its growth numbers. It was as if it was his business! Pete was always so pleased. And he had written in his last entry in his journal on January 25, the night before his second brain surgery, "I hope I make it! I would like somewhat longer to help at church." It always surprised me that church was the reason Pete would ask God for more time. He didn't ask for more time to be with me, or to work longer at the Angus Group. It must have been the most important thing to Pete. I am not sure why. Perhaps it was what he thought he'd be leaving unfinished.

Other times during Pete's hospital stay, he talked of guns and expressed a confused and generalized fear. He had asked my sister Beth to leave the hospital, because he was afraid she was going to be shot. Bill had communicated with Pete's unconscious, and Pete's unconscious told Bill that he felt God had forsaken him.

I talked to God about Pete's depression. It was terrifying for me. Pete had always been so positive in his outlook. He was the one with a "No Whining" sign on his desk at work. He was the guy who never complained, and took responsibility to always look for the positive in any situation. He rarely criticized anyone or anything. Was his positive spirit gone? Was the tumor doing this to him? Was it the medicine? Who was this man that now begged me to end it all?

Most of our friends and family thought Pete had good reason to be depressed. I realized that they, without explicitly saying so, had pretty much given up on him. The medical staff also seemed to think that things were over for Pete. They thought that I was being pretty Pollyannaish in my hope in Pete's recovery. Everyone, that is, but Nan and Bill. I would cling to Bill's visits because he helped me hope. He'd tell me that he could see God present in Pete's energy fields. A God who loved Pete very much, and sent angels regularly to help him in his battle. Nan and Bill believed with me in the possibility of Pete's healing.

One morning when praying, I felt like I hit a breakthrough about Pete's depression. Maybe God was speaking. I don't know. I didn't hear a voice. But I was inspired. I called out in the early morning darkness, "I believe in you, Pete!" I continued in my journal.

> *God has not abandoned you, Pete. I believe in Bill's message. God is with you. And you are beautiful to behold! God's spirit within you is bigger than this awful disease. I believe in you. God's spirit within your soul is more powerful than the tumor; more powerful than the weakness and confusion. You can!*
>
> *How I have failed you, Pete. I was fearful and my fear made me critical and judgmental, pushing you and fighting you over treatment or medicines. I am sorry. Please forgive me. I admire you so. How courageous you have been on this journey. Making hard decisions. Taking risks. Writing those hard notes of good-bye. How I respect you for the battle you are waging. The effort it takes you to tie your shoes and take a step. That is courage, my friend. You are so much stronger than me. I am the lucky one to be given the chance to serve you and care for you.*
>
> *I asked God to drive out the demons Pete was now facing: despair, misery, boredom, fear and shame. Give him hope in you, God, I prayed.*

Pete's Carepage: March 6, 2006 @ 9:13 p.m.

Pete made it today—the whole day without oxygen. The antibiotics have been stopped, so he continues to make progress on the pneumonia. The next step is to move him off the "heart monitoring" floor of the hospital to the "rehab" floor to get some intense therapy—physical/occupational and cognitive/speech—to build his strength so he can come home. The rehab floor move should be tomorrow. His appetite still has not come back, so that is an obstacle to his recovering. Pray now for his strength to rebuild and his eating. He is barely walking—just a few steps from the chair to his bed-and with such effort! He is brave and courageous. We thank each of you for the lift of love you give us. We feel it every day—every hour—and you sustain us through the Lord's presence.

On the seventh day of radiation treatments, Pete got off antibiotics and the rehabilitation doctor agreed to accept Pete onto the rehabilitation floor, the last stop before heading home. Pete had been in the hospital now for ten days. By day twelve, he was off the IVs and taking all his medications by mouth. Appetite was still a problem. Dr. Albright said he was getting about forty-six percent of the calorie intake he needed, and twenty-three percent of protein needed. Pete did not want the feeding tube re-inserted. I was afraid of just that.

Bill encouraged Pete to accept the feeding tube. That made me think maybe God saw the feeding tube as the best way to get Pete strong. I prayed to get over my fear of inserting the tube, and I prayed that God would find a way to make Pete want to eat. Pete grumbled, but agreed to accept the tube tomorrow. But he never had to! Another prayer answered! The rehabilitation doctor ordered megace, an appetite stimulant, instead, and Pete immediately started eating a little more. How thankful I was for our rehabilitation doctor. She made a huge difference for us.

Pete continued being very belligerent at the hospital. He didn't want to cooperate with the nurses in taking his medicine or having his vital signs taken. Pete told me "The medicine is poison."

I don't think that he wanted to keep going. He said he didn't. He felt so miserable; he just wanted it to be over. "I feel like an idiot," Pete told me.

I'd laugh at him. "Oh, you are just now figuring that out!" I'd say.

All the while I was quaking on the inside. I'd be praying quietly in my heart: *Lord, drive these demons from Pete. Help him see you as his source of hope. Help him embrace the life you have for him now.* "You are the path."

Pete responded well to therapy. He had seven appointments a day. One day he did some stairs! He did a shower on his own! Shaved himself another day! His vision had returned and tested at 20/25. The only major problem still was speech and reading. He was great with numbers, poor with words. I wondered and worried. Would Pete always be confused? Would his communication always be spotty at best? Would he ever have the strength to do the basic functions? Would we ever be able to have an adult conversation? Will he beat his depression and ever enjoy living again?

We got a home pass for the weekend. Home during the day, then back to the hospital at night. We had lunch and dinner at our table. Pete used his walker and wheelchair in the house on Saturday. By Sunday, he walked without the walker, and managed to go up the seven steps to the bathroom. Really, really took an effort. What bravery! He wanted me to get rid of the bedside commode in the living room.

We talked about how we would need to work together, and not fight each other about his care. He seemed more surrendering than ever before. For the first time in a long time, Pete picked up his beloved *Wall Street Journal* and his *Boating* and *Auto Week* magazines and showed an interest.

By the end of the following week, we stopped counting calories. His platelet counts were steadily, although slowly, improving. I got instructions from the therapists about going home: "Try to keep him from holding on to things when he walks. Keep his arms at his side. Do speech exercise half hour a day. Get him to do all the normal stuff: dishes; clothes; meal preparation. Give one-and-a-half to two hours for showering and dressing."

We got the okay to go home on March 16. "Let's get the hell out of here!" Pete said.

Dr. Albright told me, "I think he'll be back in the hospital soon. But we will let him go home for now."

Mary Jo and Mike helped me get Pete into the car at the hospital. I was so excited. On the drive home, Pete told us he wanted to go out for lunch. We looked at each other, a little surprised.

"Okay, great," Mike said. Mike was driving. "Where?"

I looked at Pete. He was silent-searching for a name.

"How about the Mount Adams Bar and Grill," I said, a favorite lunch spot of Pete's in our neighborhood. Pete smiled a yes.

I was a little afraid, but to the bar and grill it was! Pete and his amazing self. We had a great lunch, full of celebration and a beer in honor of St. Patrick's Day. Halfway through the lunch, it dawned on me that if Pete had to use the bathroom we were in trouble, because the bathroom was down a flight of twenty stairs that were steep and dark. Even if we could get him down them, we'd never get him back up. But I didn't say a word, and he didn't need to use the bathroom. But it was a good first lesson for me about casing restaurants' facilities before we made a date!

Pete's Carepage: March 17, 2006 @ 1:45 p.m.

Happy St. Patrick's Day! We are home—whoo-hoo! Got out of the hospital yesterday afternoon and Pete was feeling so good he asked to go out to lunch. So Mike and Mary Jo and Pete and I had lunch at the Mount Adams Bar & Grill! Very cool! Who would have thought? Thanks to each of you for your continued prayers.

Our routine now is radiation treatments Monday through Friday. On Tuesdays and Thursdays Pete will have physical, speech and occupational therapy after radiation at the hospital. On the "off days" we do exercises at home. We are about half way through radiation treatments so we have about another month of those. Pete still needs twenty-four-hour care, but at least now we can be together in our own home. Nice to sleep together again!

Feels like another milestone to me and Pete! What a journey this has been, and we are far from over. You are so faithful to us—checking these Carepages so many times and sending messages and cards of encouragement and prayer. This afternoon, I am going to help Pete get current on all of your messages. He'll love that! And we will both get a boost of energy! Love and gratitude to all.

While Pete was in the hospital, I had asked Mike to go into our house, find Pete's guns, and store them at his house for awhile. Pete loved guns and had used them at target ranges, and had occasionally gone hunting with Steve. I was fearful enough about Pete's depression. I didn't want to make it easy for him to have an accident. I also asked Mike and Mary Jo if they would be willing to make a trip to Spring Grove cemetery and pick out a plot for Pete. The only criteria were that the plot had to be on a hill and have a southern exposure. The sun always needed to be in Pete's face.

Pete had told me he wanted to be buried in Spring Grove, but we had never taken the next step. Would they be willing? Just in case Pete didn't recover. I gave them the names of the people Pete had placed at Spring Grove through his recruiting relationship. Spring Grove was one of his clients, and he had placed the CEO, the president and a few others. When Mike and Mary Jo went to visit, they were treated like royalty! All the staff showed such love for Pete! And they found a couple of plots they thought would do just fine. But thankfully, we ended up not needing them then!

Pete was getting better. He still slept a lot during the day. I had to push him to do his exercises, take a shower or shave. We turned our den upstairs into our bedroom, because it only required eight steps to our living area versus sixteen steps if we had gone down to our master bedroom and bath. We slept on the fold-out bed in the sofa.

Pete was sent home with a walker, which he used when we were outside the house. He walked more and more independently inside. On the second day home, Pete walked with his walker and me at his side up our street, which has a very San Francisco-type grade. It took two and a half hours to make a half block, but he made it. Each day we would mark our progress with a mini-celebration.

"Made the stairs on your own!" I'd exclaim one day.

"Took a shower standing up!" warranted a "whoo-hoo!"

"Got on and off the toilet without my help today!"

"You are walking more and more on your own. Your balance is getting better," I'd say as I high-fived him.

One day after our visitors left, I looked at him with delight and said, "You are amazing; the consummate gentleman! Our guests are here to visit you, the sick one, but you are the one who stands up, shakes their hand, and walks them to the door! How I love you!" I said as I kissed and hugged him.

Our lives were returning to a new normal. By the sixth day after Pete was home, he went to the grocery store with me. I was as excited as if it was our first date. We had lots of firsts within those first ten days home. I cheered Pete on. We were like kids on a team that was winning the tournament, one game after another. Marking the milestones toward recovery was important.

My prayer journal: March 7, 2006

I've put Pete in your hands. I can't heal him. I can't fix him. Take good care of him, Lord. He needs your protection in his weakened state. Drive out Satan and his evil powers. You are bigger. You have conquered Satan. You have conquered evil. May your warrior angels keep doing their work in Pete. You are the path out of Pete's desire to end it all. When I asked you what to do with Pete's request, you answered me. "Do not judge. Understand his pain and misery. Understand his fear. Understand his weariness. Don't be afraid of his depression. His hopelessness. I am your path. I will lead you out." Help him want to eat, Lord.

It is terrifying to me, Lord, to be in this decision-making role for Pete. I don't want it. I don't know what you are doing with him or what you want. Show us the right way to navigate this medical system. Help me be an advocate as necessary. To discover your will for Pete. You are bigger than me. So I rest in the knowledge that you will do for Pete. You will act. You will heal him-spiritually-physically-mentally and emotionally. I ask for your healing power, your Holy Spirit, your angels to invade Pete. And I surrender him—surrender us—to you. May your Holy Spirit guide me in this hospital world. It is such a terrifying world. Pete is so sick. May your healing presence guide the hospital staff and your love guide their care of him. Where you lead, I will follow.

11
Recovery

I marked Pete's recovery from the brain tumor surgeries and pneumonia by our first overnight trip away from home that wasn't to a hospital. It was a short little trip to the Glen Laurel Lodge in Hocking Hills Park in southeastern Ohio, just two and a half hours away from home. It was the last day of April, 2006. Pete's brain surgery had occurred on January 17, 2006. Here's the story of his recovery.

Diarrhea was Pete's constant companion, and a complication that would create suffering for him through his whole journey. He would have attacks multiple times a day, and then be exhausted and have to rest. My heart broke for him each time. Although he never said anything or complained about it, the threat of a diarrhea attack must have been a source of constant anxiety for him. All the more amazing, that during this time, Pete would still get out for meetings and have dinner with friends!

We finally visited an intestinal specialist, and he diagnosed Pete with a C-diff infection, which is typically gotten when in the hospital for a long stay, especially when taking antibiotics. The hospital had tested Pete for this infection a number of times while he was hospitalized, and the results had always been negative. But either the tests were wrong or the samples poor, because Pete had C-diff. To treat it, Pete had to take the medicine Flagyl, which killed the C-diff infection. He couldn't drink any alcohol when he was on Flagyl, or he'd get deathly sick. One of Pete's hobbies was wine. He had educated himself (and me) about wine over the last ten years. Giving up his daily glass of wine just didn't seem fair after all he had been through!

Flagyl was a medication that was scheduled to taper, with lighter doses following heavier ones. Each cycle lasted about two weeks. Pete ended up having to go through two full cycles of Flagyl. After he finished the first cycle toward the end of March, we rejoiced! But within days of stopping the medicine, the diarrhea returned and we had to start all over again. In fact, Pete's diarrhea attack had gotten in the way initially of our trip to Glen Laurel. We had to cancel. But we rescheduled for the following week, and what a time we had!

Periodically, Pete would still fight me about taking his medications. "It's poison," Pete would say to me.

I'd get really mad. "Do you think you are smarter than the doctors?" I'd ask.

He would sit in silence, but adamant about not taking his pills which were sitting in my open hand, in front of his face. When I talked to Steve about it, he said, "Dad doesn't want to take his medicine, because he knows it is hopeless. He is going to die and his medicine just prolongs it."

My heart felt crushed, as I listened to Steve's words.

I'd look at Pete and, with all the force of my will, I'd lecture him: "It's my responsibility to make sure you get your medicine. I don't give you anything that is not necessary. I even eliminate some of the less important pills. This is my job as a caregiver. I am not going to let you get away with not taking your medicine. If you won't take the medicine, maybe you need to get another caregiver. It's your choice. Now what do you want to do?" I'd say.

I hated those exchanges. And so did Pete. He began to look at me with dread. I felt such anguish knowing we had such little time together, and we were spending it in anger. "Oh, I don't want to screw this up," I'd sigh.

Pete would roll his eyes when telling Mike about our conversations. "Really bad today," Pete would tell Mike after one of our battles.

I didn't know what to do. I felt helpless. Was it my own selfishness that kept driving me so strongly? Was it love of Pete? Was it compliance with the doctors and fear to disobey? We were both very strong-willed people, and Pete's medicines were putting us to the test. I didn't know how much longer I could go on with these intense battles. I knew I was causing the problem, and I criticized myself mercilessly for doing something wrong and not being able to see it.

I agreed to try to eliminate any unnecessary medications. It was always a topic during each doctor's visit. I called Dr. Albright's office one day when Pete's resistance was really strong, to ask them if they could eliminate any of the medicines now. They said they didn't want to do it until they saw him for the next visit, which was in a few days. That seemed to satisfy Pete. We had gone on record with the doctor!

Pete was right in some of his resistance to his medicines. Doctors never told you to stop taking anything after they initially prescribed it. The numbers of pills just kept adding up. When Pete pushed, sometimes he won!

About two weeks after Pete got home from the hospital, we sat at the computer and he talked while I typed in a message to all of our followers on the Carepages. His eyes got misty, as he thought about what he wanted to say. He was so touched by the number of messages, and all the people who showed their care and faithfulness to him. He wanted a short message.

Pete's Carepage: March 26, 2006 @ 5:13 p.m.

I am so happy to see all your messages. I have read them all and am amazed at how many of you have stuck with me through all of this. Thank you. I am a little sore from falling yesterday. Thank goodness we have carpet where we are sleeping. Don't think it is serious—don't have much feeling on my right side—but doesn't look like anything is broken. It has been great to be at home this last week. Most days have been good ones. I am still very weak. Steve from DC came in today, and Kathy and I picked him up from the airport and stopped for lunch at Skyline Chili, our tradition when he comes into town. I was able to walk into Skyline and maybe we will do ribs tonight at Montgomery Inn. It's important to have fun!

§ § § § §

One Response:

Hey Pete and Kathy,
    Keep on fighting. You are making progress in so many ways. The two of you together are generating a huge amount of power, not only for your lives but in the lives of hundreds of others! God is with you! Jeannie and I continue to pray with you.

Tim

The next weeks were full of good days and sleepy days. I was monitoring Pete's blood sugar, which stayed on the low side. His blood pressure was coming into the normal range, after we stopped taking any blood pressure medicine at all. We didn't ask any doctor for permission to stop the blood pressure medicine. We had been monitoring Pete's blood pressure so closely, and it had been in the low range for so long, we just decided to stop. One less medicine for Pete to take! That ended up being the right decision, since any dizziness or balance issues disappeared shortly thereafter. Since losing all that weight, Pete just didn't need the blood pressure medication. It was the only time I remember doing something medical without a doctor's approval.

Pete's platelet count moved to eighty-four thousand. A one hundred thousand count would allow Pete to take Temodar, the chemotherapy agent that would make his radiation more effective. Diarrhea was still a challenge, but Pete's strength was definitely improving. We still slept upstairs in the office, but he was making it downstairs for breakfast and back up the eight stairs for dressing, showering and shaving. He started to walk more and more without a walker. Pete fell a couple of times. Each time was scary for him and me. He fell once in the bedroom, when he got up to go to the bathroom early one morning, and once at a restaurant when he missed the top step. We were blessed because nothing was broken, and we both learned the value of being cautious.

Pete went to Joe's Crab Shack with Mary Jo and Mike for dinner without me, while I was doing a video for a bank event. They had a great time and Pete loved his clam soup. Pete trimmed his own moustache. He reviewed the taxes with me. He longed for a day with no schedule.

Saturdays—how awesome they were! As April came he told me, "Life has changed significantly but I kind of like this! No work!"

Pete had changed. I was learning more as we spent time together at home. He now had a relaxed attitude about things that used to be a source of upset. A great example of this change was the day I hit another car. He was in the passenger seat. I was pulling up to the hospital entrance for his radiation treatment number twenty-five. I was driving Pete's car. His beloved BMW M3! It was Friday afternoon. I hit the driver side door of a hospital worker's car when I was backing up. It was just a little bump, but it was due to my carelessness. Pete was very calm. He didn't get angry as he would have normally over an incident like that. Since it was a small repair, neither of us wanted to use our insurance to pay for it. In prior times, Pete might have resisted paying her repair bill, or made sure she had at least two estimates so he was assured we weren't being taken advantage of. But not this time. Things just weren't as earth-shattering to him now as they had been before all this.

Lots of little things gave us such pleasure. Nan and Bill invited us to go out to dinner on a Saturday night. We chose one of our old favorite Italian restaurants, Barresi's. Pete walked very slowly, but he walked with a cane on his own, into the restaurant. How he loved dining out, and how he loved Italian food. We got such pleasure in remembering all the dinners we had enjoyed there with our two sons for special occasions.

Then one night, Mary Jo and Mike came over while Steve was visiting and we cooked together at our house. Pete's favorite—salmon on the grill! What a great time we had, with everyone pitching in and cooking together. What joy was in our dining room that night! The love between each of us filled our house!

Then one afternoon, we were alone in our living room and a Kenny Rogers song played on the radio. Pete moved toward me without saying a word. He put his arm around me and we slow-danced together. Just spontaneous! He held me so gently. The love in his eyes for me was deep and precious. I felt like the most beautiful girl in the world.

Pete's Carepage: March 30, 2006 @ 7:53 p.m.

We had a good day! Last night and today Mary Jo joined us and we saw three docs: Pete's primary care, the radiologist and Dr A, our oncologist. Pete's mission was to get as many pills ditched as possible. Last night we got the primary care doc to ditch the blood sugar pill which means Pete's blood sugar spike, caused by the steroids is definitely going in the right direction, and he doesn't need medication for it anymore! The radiologist was very encouraged by Pete's progress. The "grit" part of the radiation treatment is now upon us, since the radiation effect is cumulative in its impact, and we just finished treatment #24 of 33 treatments. The radiologist was surprised at the level of Pete's stamina and speech. The radiation is starting to affect Pete's hearing and his saliva glands (both temporary) due to the location of the treatment so the radiologist added a pill (boo!) to help Pete's appetite, but he only has to take it for seven days. Yeah! And if it works—it's worth it. Dr A, the oncologist, got rid of four pills! Whoo-hoo! Which means Pete's blood counts, his potassium, appetite and nutrition profile are all headed in the right direction. Dr A had told me two weeks ago that he expected Pete back in the hospital by now, just because of the radiation impact on his already weak body. Delighted us no end to NOT be in the hospital AND to have Dr A eliminate some medications. So thank goodness for Bill and his healing touch work with Pete every day after radiation treatments to lessen the negative impact. Thank goodness for all—and each—of you who have been praying for Pete's appetite and his strength and endurance to improve. Thank God for all of you and the wonder of His work.

Pete was reading more. The thought of buying a new car had now captured his imagination. He was reading his *Car and Driver, Auto Week* and *BMW Excellence* magazines again. Pete had always loved car shopping. In the past, he would spend months looking by himself, and then take me with him on many a Saturday and Sunday afternoon. It was entertainment for Pete. We currently owned a 2000 Porsche 911 we had bought at the factory in Stuttgart, Germany, and a BMW-M3 sports car. I drove the Porsche and Pete drove the M3. Both were convertibles. Neither car made it easy for Pete to get in and out. Neither could hold a wheelchair easily.

We had decided it was time to buy something a little more in line with our new life. Pete watched cars on the road when we were out, and asked me what I liked when he saw one he was attracted to. We were thinking an SUV, or maybe a cross-over of some sort. Neither of us liked big cars.

We went car shopping and asked Mike to come along after we had narrowed our choices down to either an Audi 4 wagon, a Mercedes SUV, or a BMW sports wagon. Pete used his cane when we walked the car lots. I took the wheelchair with us to test the hatchbacks ease of access. What a funny trio we were. We had a blast.

Pete made the decision easily after we had test-driven each of the cars. We went back to the BMW store and negotiated a deal on a new sports wagon by trading in his BMW M3. They did a computer search for a car with our desired specifications. It was located in Pennsylvania, and would be ours in a few weeks. Pete was so excited!

On Monday, April 3, 2006, we went in to the hospital vascular lab for a precautionary Doppler test, to make sure Pete didn't have any blood clots. Pete's ankles were a little swollen, which led me to bring the topic up with the doctor. He never had any pain or redness in his legs or ankles, but to be safe, Dr. Albright ordered a Doppler exam.

The technician doing the Doppler used a wand about the size of a small vacuum cleaner head. Cold goop was heated, and spread on Pete's legs. By moving the wand over this goop on Pete's legs, a picture was displayed on the computer screen. I could see the pulsating blood through Pete's veins on the computer. The technician taught me how to identify a clot on the screen. She looked at us with compassion and simply said, "You won't be leaving here, today." I was so discouraged.

I called Bill, who was scheduled to come to our home within the hour to do Pete's daily healing touch treatment. Instead, Bill came to the Doppler lab at the hospital. Bill's presence was a blessing. He did Healing Touch on Pete while in the hall of the Doppler Lab.

Pete's Carepage: April 3, 2006 @ 10:58 p.m.

This is Mike & Mary Jo. Unfortunately, we just left Pete and Kathy at Good Samaritan Hospital where Pete has been re-admitted. Pete has had some swelling in his ankles and he had a test this afternoon for blood clots. Unfortunately, multiple clots were found in both legs and Pete was admitted to the hospital. The current plan is to start Pete on blood thinner tonight. As soon as possible a filter will be inserted into Pete's vein that comes from his legs to catch any blood clots that try to move. Kathy requests that we send special prayers that the clots stay put until they are dissolved or until the filter is inserted. Other than blood clots, Pete continues to improve. His speech continues to progress and his spirits are good. Pete and Kathy went out to dinner Saturday night with Nan and Bill. They also attended services at Crossroads on Sunday. Our hope is that this is a temporary setback and that we can get Pete home again shortly. As we left the hospital tonight, the last thing Kathy asked is that we update the Carepages so your special prayers can begin. Your prayers and support make all the difference to Pete and Kathy.

Blood clots came with brain tumors. No one knows why, but there was a high incidence of them. Pete was confined to bed rest for the next four to five days. He could get up only to use the bedside commode. They took him on a stretcher to continue his radiation treatments. Pete's diarrhea came back. He had two accidents the first night he was in the hospital, and subsequent bowel movements at nine a.m., and at one-thirty, six and seven-thirty p.m. When was he going to get some relief?!

One of the safeguards that Dr. Albright used to protect brain tumor patients from blood clots was to put a filter in the vena cava, where the two large veins from each leg join just below the belly button. The purpose of the filter was to catch any clot that might dislodge from either leg and move toward a more important organ, such as the heart or lungs. The filter was permanent. It was placed by a radiologist in a surgical procedure. Before Pete could get the filter inserted, he needed platelet transfusions to ensure that he wouldn't bleed to death when the filter was inserted. By Wednesday afternoon, the filter was inserted and all went smoothly. I was thankful to God for protecting Pete through this procedure.

The culture on Pete's stool showed positive for C-Diff again—so back to the Flagyl medicine. Ugh! We had a scare during this stay because Pete's white blood cell count dropped significantly and fast. Why? Bone marrow production being obstructed somehow? A day later the count appeared stable. No real answers. The roller-coaster ride continued. But by Friday afternoon, April 7, we were home!

At home, Pete walked down the stairs and into the garage on his own. He walked into a restaurant near the hospital for lunch—on his own! He sat outside on the deck. He managed to get himself into the hammock for a nap in the sun. He cut oranges and squeezed us fresh orange juice for breakfast. He cut the meat and soaked the peas over-night for pea soup, and made the best soup he had ever made! The diarrhea was slowing. Spring was coming!

Two days before Pete's radiation treatments were over, Pete walked into the radiation department on his own. No wheelchair or walker! He was like a triumphant soldier coming back from the war! How proud he was, and how proud I was of him. The radiation staff let out a whoop and holler. "Look what we got here!" they joyously exclaimed.

Pete's Carepage: April 13, 2006 @ 9:12 p.m.

SPRING HAS DEFINITELY LIFTED OUR SPIRITS! So beautiful to see the world come anew again and to enjoy a little sunshine out-side on our deck. Pete even lit the grill for the first time in months yes-terday! Oh, the little, normal things! I asked him if the fire was ready for the lamb chops and he said "Not really. It's still cold. Don't know what is wrong." I walked outside and the coals looked hot to me, so I put my hand over them and felt the heat. "What makes you think it is not ready?" I asked. "Use your left hand to test it," I said. Immedi-ately Pete jumped back from the heat. He didn't feel the heat at all with his right hand. Good lesson for him and me!

Radiation is OVER! The staff actually gave Pete a "graduation" certificate. How wonderful the radiology staff has been to us at Good Sam. They have walked this journey the whole six weeks with us and have loved Pete all along the way. BIG milestone! Thanks for all of you who have been praying for a successful completion.

We also visited Dr A. today and he was surprised at how well Pete was doing. Pete actually walked into the doc office today with only a cane, which was a first! We will know the impact of the radiation treatments at the next MRI which is scheduled for May 4. We should get a picture of what is happening with the tumor then. But the good news is Pete is gaining weight. He gained four pounds to a robust 144! His white blood counts are okay and most other measures are all trending positive! His speech therapist says he has improved almost fifty percent based on her assessment this week. His strength in his hands has also improved by thirty-three percent! And Bill and Nan, our healing touch friends, have found the archangels—Michael, Raphael and Uriel—all with Pete now for the last couple of days. So God does send his warriors (and the best ones, at that!) to do battle for us.

Focus now on asking God to dissolve the blood clots in Pete's legs and to build his strength. His protein levels are still way too low despite all the "force feeding" I am doing. (God help us—me cooking!) And the low protein levels aggravate the swelling in his ankles and feet because the blood cells can't absorb all the water and the extra fluid settles in the lowest point.

How we count on you! Your prayers and support continue to lead us through and lift us with whatever we need: hope, strength, sleep and these days—a little joy! Thank you!

April 17, 2006, marked ninety short days from two brain surgeries, ninety-six hours of IL-13 infusions, thirty-three radiation treatments, a bad case of pneumonia, seven blood clots and chronic diarrhea. Pete never looked back. The depression and despair he had felt in February and March totally disappeared. I mean, like poof! Gone. Not gradually, getting better over several weeks. But totally gone. He never expressed any depression or sad feelings again. It was impossible for me to imagine that just a few weeks ago he had begged me to end it all. The nightmare was over. It was amazing. I don't know if it was the change in his medicines, or Bill's Healing Touch, or God's driving out Pete's demons, or just the normal recovery process, but Pete started to really enjoy life again. I stopped worrying as much, and we started to have a blast. I don't think I was ever happier in our relationship as I was right then.

Pete typed this update himself as we sat down at the computer at home in mid-April of 2006.

Pete's Carepage: April 19, 2006 @ 8:29 p.m.

This is Pete! Thank you all very much for your notes and messages. They are very effective to me. I appreciate your personal encouragement and I respond to them with positive feelings. Everything is getting better—body and mind. I am doing things like—I smoked my favorite ribs in my "smoker" tonight and swept out the garage. But I am still working on getting my legs working right—they are still swollen and very weak. I can't walk or stand very long. So I look forward to the future and count on your support and prayers.

P.S. This is Kathy. Our BIG project since the last update was buying a new car. Pete researched alternatives for days—the best speech therapy he could ever get! He was passionate about looking and studying! Steve tried to talk him into changing his sports car for a minivan. Pete just nodded his head to that suggestion. But we knew two two-seater convertibles were not the most practical for wheelchairs or guys with canes. So we finally decided to trade in the BMW M3 for a station wagon. Now it is a nice station wagon—they call it a "BMW 325xi sports wagon" and it doesn't drive bad at all, and it has a BIG moon roof for front and back seats and can handle a wheelchair without a problem and is low enough for Pete to get into it, but not so low that he feels like he is crawling out. We're excited— another change in our "new" life. Good-bye M3—we loved you so!

We got our new car the last day of April, and by the next day we were on our way to the Hocking Hills of Ohio to spend the night at the Glen Laurel Lodge. Pete navigated while I drove the new car. How excited we were. Pete wrote in a letter to a good friend later, "I am feeling pretty well and for the first time have been able to make a one night trip with wife Kathy. We drove our new car and it was pretty neat."

The Glen Laurel Lodge was a Scottish inn nestled in the crevice of the hills in southeast Ohio. It was still chilly at the end of April in Ohio, and as we pulled up we could see the smoke from the fireplace against the backdrop of blooming fruit trees. As he got out of the car, Pete leaned against the hood of his new car, and I snapped a picture.

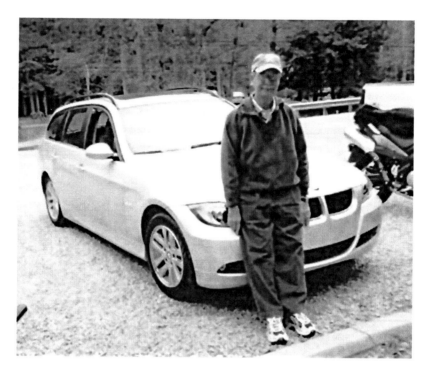

Pete in front of his new car at Glen Laurel Lodge

Our room was on the first floor so we had no steps to conquer. The lodge was small, twelve rooms. The hosts of the lodge invited all the guests to join them for a happy hour on the outside stone deck before dinner. I wasn't too interested in going. But Pete, the ever-social gentleman, wouldn't miss it. So here was our first night away from home, and we walked into a gathering of people who we didn't know and who didn't know us. Pete did not use a cane. He walked right up to greet people and shook their hands, just like he was at a chamber meeting or some professional gathering he had gone to a million times before he had brain cancer. He didn't use his or my name in the introductions. I stayed close by his side. The conversation jumped around to where we were from, and what we did for a living, and the weather, and the outlook for the Reds baseball team. Pete smiled and talked even though all the words didn't come out exactly right. He didn't show any self-consciousness. I couldn't believe Pete's confidence and ease in talking to all the lodge guests. I'd fill in a word for him now and then when he was searching for it. I don't think any of the guests suspected Pete had just had brain surgery. I was beaming with pride, and he was almost strutting as the lodge staff led us into the dining room for a sumptuous seven-course dinner.

That night, with a fire blazing in the fireplace in our room, Pete got interested in sex for the first time since surgery. I knew then that his recovery was complete! The next day, we went on two handicap-accessible hiking trails in the beautiful woods. I laughed as Pete pushed his empty wheelchair up the trails. He was so determined not to use the wheelchair. He wanted to walk as long and as far as he could on his own. Such a thrill being in the woods and exploring the caves! We rested regularly, the empty wheelchair parked beside us.

12

Medications and Healing Touch

Medications.

I came to learn that the big problem with a malignant brain tumor was not the tumor itself; many can be surgically removed. The problem was the brain cancer cells that stay alive in and around the bed where the original tumor was. Those cancer cells, although not able to be seen, are alive. These brain cancer cells will continue to grow, invade brain tissue, and become a brain tumor when they become big enough to be visible. That's what a recurrent brain tumor is. For a high-grade glioblastoma multiforme tumor like Pete had, the recurrence rate is very high. Almost all of the treatment for brain tumor patients, whether radiation, chemotherapy, Avastin or treatments being tested in various clinical trials, was an attempt to kill those invisible brain cancer cells so that the brain tumor would not recur.

Pete was on two medications for treating his brain cancer: steroids and anti-seizure medication. Neither of these medications did anything to prevent the tumor from recurring. Pete was prescribed anti-seizure medications from the very first day we saw the very first doctor, when they diagnosed Pete with a brain tumor.

"About thirty to forty percent of patients with brain tumors will have a seizure (involuntary movements, twitching or being 'out of it' for moments to minutes) at one time or another. This has practical implications for employment, driving, and overall independence.

115

Anticonvulsants reduce the chance of having another seizure. Anti-seizure medications tone down the electrical activity in the brain that sets off the seizure."

—*Brain Tumors: Leaving the Garden of Eden.*

There were a lot of different types of anti-seizure medications. Pete took Dilantin, Depakote, Keppra and Topamax at different times. The doctor finally settled on Topamax, and Pete would take fifty mg. in the morning and fifty mg. in the evening. For patients who have frequent seizures, the dosage can be as high as three thousand mg. a day. Pete had only one seizure during his whole illness, and that was immediately after his first surgery. But the fear was always there.

The anti-seizure medication had an effect on Pete's platelet counts, which was why the doctors kept switching medications. They were trying to find the medication with the least negative impact. Other than that, the anti-seizure medications just made Pete drowsy. It was not unusual for Pete to nap for a short while right after taking his morning medications, and I think the anti-seizure medicine was the major reason.

Steroids control swelling and inflammation in the brain. "Dexamethasone/Decadron is the most powerful type of manufactured steroid and mimics the function of bodily-produced cortisol." When taking steroids, Pete's body stopped producing cortisol, which was a natural hormone produced by his adrenal gland. "The body's total daily production of cortisol is equivalent of .75 mg. of Decadron. 12 mg. of Decadron is sixteen times as much as normally made in your body," according to *Brain Tumors: Leaving the Garden of Eden.*

Right after surgery, Pete was on twenty-four mg. of Decadron. He had doses in the twenty mg. range for a long time after surgery. Pete finally settled in between two to four mg. of Decadron a day along with an antacid, which was standard when taking a steroid, to offset the irritation the drug gave to his gastrointestinal system. This seemed to be the minimal dose required for Pete to provide a positive effect. If Pete had stopped taking Decadron without any tapering he would have had serious physical consequences, since the body needed to restart making its own cortisol before he stopped taking the medication. Steroids were the medicine that Pete seemed to respond to the best in his recovery.

There is nothing good about steroids. It did bad stuff to Pete's body. I had memorized the chapters in all the medical guides about the side effects of steroid use, from re-reading them so many times.

We always wondered whether the IL-13 treatment actually created some inflammation in Pete's brain that the steroids somehow controlled, and gave Pete such positive effect. We will never know. However, when Pete was on steroids his speech was better, his thinking more clear and focused, and his sense of humor enhanced. (Just kidding.) Pete probably got dependent on steroids. I remember a few days before we were getting ready to leave for our trip to France to see the 24 Heures du Mans when Pete started complaining of bad headaches. Pete had never had a headache through this whole ordeal! But all of sudden he had a headache. He was on a tapering schedule to get off of the steroids, and was just about ready to start his first day without any. A quick call to Dr. Albright, and Pete's taper was discontinued and he was back to a low dosage.

The clinic told us that the steroids kept having a positive effect on the inflammation in Pete's brain tissue. When he was on steroids at a high enough level, the MRI would show that the enhancements were much less pronounced or actually shrank; when he was decreasing the steroid dosage, the enhancements actually grew. Dr. Albright hated the impact of the steroids on Pete, and told us many times of the damaging effects the steroids were having and would have on Pete's health in the long term. Those effects included osteoporosis leading to fractures, kidney stones, diabetes, and all kinds of susceptibility to infections.

The steroids took their toll on Pete. The muscles in his upper thighs were getting eaten away by the steroids. He experienced weakness in his legs, especially when climbing steps or getting up from a chair. It was visible. I could see his thighs losing their muscle mass. As skinny as his thighs got, the bigger his abdomen, the cheeks in his face and his ankles got. Steroids made him hold fluids and this fluid settled in the lowest point in his body, which was his ankles. A footstool became a permanent fixture near Pete's chair, and he'd raise his legs whenever he was sitting. We also got some support hose which Pete wore especially at the later stages, when his vanity was just not important to him anymore.

The steroids also acted as a stimulant to Pete's appetite. He went from a low weight of one hundred and thirty-seven pounds in March of 2006 to pushing two hundred pounds by September of 2007. The weight gain was centered in his abdomen. We had to shop for new pants and jeans, since Pete's waist size had increased by six inches. Pete hated getting heavy. He resisted getting new pants and belts as long as he could.

Pete's skin also became paper-thin. It was not unusual for him to have Band-Aids on his arms and hands in several spots. Any small bump would cause bleeding. The arm of his favorite chair had bloodstains on the arm protectors. I carried Band-Aids in my wallet, so if he started bleeding while we were out I was ready. The steroids also increased Pete's blood sugar levels, creating what the doctors call "steroid-induced diabetes." Regular monitoring of Pete's blood sugar became part of our daily routine. At its worst point, I needed to prick Pete's fingers four times a day to test his blood sugar. His poor fingers. He dreaded it, and so did I. At times the high blood sugar required additional medications, ranging from a dose of glucophage to injections of insulin.

The standard treatment for brain tumor patients was surgery and six weeks of radiation with Temodar, an oral chemotherapy. These standard treatments were meant to reduce the chance of the brain tumor recurring. Pete completed radiation, but he never took Temodar during the radiation because of his low platelet blood count. The reason he participated in the IL-13 clinical trial was to prevent his tumor from recurring by killing those hidden brain cancer cells. Some form of additional chemotherapy or experimental treatments would be used if the tumor did recur. Patients and caregivers live in constant vigilance and uncertainty.

There were numerous alternative treatments available for people who had any form of cancer. The options were overwhelming. Pete's friend Joe, who had a brain tumor in the same place as Pete's, used acupuncture, massage, healing touch and numerous vitamin and nutritional solutions. Another friend, John, who was a ten-year brain tumor survivor, "drank green tea—lots of it," in addition to the standard treatments. "More than sixty percent of people with brain tumors and other cancers use non-traditional medications and approaches to help them feel better or fight their cancer."

In *Brain Tumors: Finding the Ark* there was a full list, and this helpful categorization.

1. Biological Therapies: Herbs and nutritional supplements; special diets; natural compounds which alleviate symptoms or control cancer.

2. Manipulative and Body-Based methods: chiropractic; osteopathic manipulations; massage; physical therapy; yoga which give symptom relief.

3. Energy Therapies: Reiki; therapeutic touch; electrical devices which give symptom relief.

4. Mind-Body Interventions: art therapies; biofeedback; hypnotherapy; meditation; psychotherapy; spiritual counseling and others practiced by healers which give symptom relief and coping.

Pete did not get involved in many of these alternative treatments. He used only one, and that was Healing Touch. Healing Touch would be categorized as an energy therapy.

In our Carepage entries we mentioned Bill, our healer, several times. Bill was a friend who, after a very successful career in banking, became a Healing Touch professional and committed Christian. I knew Bill as a former colleague at the bank. His wife Nan and I were the best of friends. Pete and I and Bill and Nan were friends before Pete got diagnosed. Our relationship got much deeper and more intimate with the onset of Pete's tumor. Bill and Nan made a commitment to walk with us on our journey. They stepped toward in us in ways neither Pete nor I would ever have imagined.

Bill and Pete shared a love of guns, hunting and making business deals. During an energy medicine assessment, it was discovered Bill had an abdominal aneurysm. This happened a couple of years before Pete got his brain tumor. Bill's aneurysm was successfully removed. A neighbor of his visited him before surgery, and did Healing Touch on Bill. Bill's recovery was much faster than anyone had anticipated. As a result, Bill became interested in Healing Touch, convinced that Healing Touch had been the reason for his amazing recovery from surgery. During his study of Healing Touch, Bill found that he actually had a gift for healing others.

Bill made a commitment to a course of study. He became a Healing Touch practitioner. He administered Healing Touch to friends and family members and to patients in hospice. Bill taught others about techniques he had developed himself. Throughout this process, Bill went through a major life change, becoming an ardent Christ-follower. Bill would tell Pete and me, "I am just a messenger of God. I just listen and obey His guidance."

On our very first doctor visit, when Pete was initially diagnosed with a brain tumor, Bill met Pete in the doctor's office parking lot afterward. Bill took Pete to a Healing Touch session. Bill had just achieved the first level of Healing Touch. Bill wanted Pete to have the best, so Bill took Pete to a healer who was a level five certified Healing Touch professional. Pete had his first experience with Healing

Touch that day. Pete asked Bill during that first visit to be his pall bearer. Bill said yes. Pete told Bill that he was advised by his doctors that he had about ninety days to live.

The second time Pete experienced Healing Touch, Bill did it himself. Bill had received a spiritual message to bring bread and wine and offer Pete "communion," which he did. Pete agreed to receive the bread and wine, and when Bill asked if Pete had accepted Christ as his Savior, Pete said yes.

Bill told me later with tears in his eyes, "In the face of death, Pete Nadherny was the bravest man I've ever met. He lived for over two years! I shall love him for all of eternity."

When Pete and I left for the Cleveland Clinic for surgery two weeks later, Bill stayed connected with Pete's energy fields. Bill worked on Pete remotely every day we were at the clinic. Bill explained that energy fields have no geographical boundaries, so if permitted, he can work on anyone in any location.

Healing Touch was one of those energy therapies listed above. Healing Touch re-aligned Pete's energy fields, which increased the energy flows in his body. Energy flows through all of our bodies. Each part of our body has a different electrical frequency of energy. A healthy body energy frequency is between sixty-two and sixty-eight megahertz. The brain has the highest frequency in the body, at seventy to ninety megahertz. Diseases have lower frequencies: colds at fifty-eight, viruses at fifty-seven and cancer at forty-two megahertz.

Healing Touch believes that all healing in the body is basically self-healing. Healing Touch practitioners complemented the self-healing process, operating from an energy perspective rather than just physical. Increasing the energy flows in the body eliminated blockages to self-healing. "During treatment, the practitioner's biomagnetic field interacts with the client's biomagnetic field and changes occur in the client's electrical field. This produces a change in the client's chemical balance at the cellular level, chemicals are released and physiological changes result. The cell's structure and function are changed."

Normally Pete would have been a little skeptical of anything that was as ethereal-sounding as Healing Touch. But in this instance, Pete showed no hesitation. He was all over it. Given his circumstances and odds, Pete tried anything that had promise to help. And Bill was Pete's friend. Pete trusted Bill.

Bill began doing Healing Touch on Pete every day except Sundays once we moved back to Cincinnati. He did these treatments in person.

He lived about thirty miles north of Cincinnati. Pete and I lived downtown. I estimated that Bill did over one hundred healing touch sessions in those months while Pete was receiving radiation and in the hospital with pneumonia. Bill drove over six thousand miles in those first critical months to heal Pete. Simultaneously, Bill continued his course of study and finished Healing Touch Level IV.

"I asked God once," Bill told me, "if I should get someone else to be Pete's healer since I lacked experience."

"What did God say?' I asked.

"He told me that he was going to work through me, and not to worry about my experience. It was my heart that mattered."

I smiled and loved Bill all the more for his innocence, integrity and love for Pete.

A Healing Touch session would go something like this. Bill would come into the house or hospital room, and we would visit for a short while. Nan came with Bill to these treatments about seventy-five percent of the time. Nan and I stayed close to Pete and Bill during the treatment. We would be praying all the while Bill was working.

Bill would give me a chart that outlined the human energy fields on a sketch of a body. I dated the chart and took notes about what Bill assessed in Pete that day, and what treatment he used. It was quiet in the room. A session would usually last between an hour to two hours.

Bill would first ask, "Pete, are you having any pain?" Pete always answered "No." Then Bill put out his hands, moving about six inches above and over Pete's body to get in sync with Pete's energy fields. He did an assessment of Pete, all the time listening for God's guidance as to where he should work that day, and where he should begin. Sometimes he would be led to drain pollutants out of Pete's energy fields. Pollutants impeded energy flow in the body. There were lots of pollutants: toxins, emotional hooks, past traumas, pain, phobias, and lack of forgiveness in our energy fields. If Pete's energy fields had pollutants, they tended to be toxins or emotional hooks. Bill explained that toxins could come from anywhere. Toxins in our society were in the air we breathed, or they could be from the radiation Pete was receiving. Emotional hooks were emotions that needed expression, and could be from current or past situations. An example of an emotional hook would be sadness.

Bill assessed where the blockages were in Pete's energy fields, and drained out those blockages. When Bill did a pollutant drain, his hand and arm would be stretched out over the energy field where the pollutant was housed in Pete. Bill's eyes would usually be closed. Sometimes his hand and arm shook uncontrollably, as the pollutants moved from Pete's energy field through Bill's arm out through his hand, and as Bill would say, "into the universe." Sometimes Bill felt a tingling, as if the toxins were burning him. There were occasions when Bill's drains would take fifteen to twenty minutes, and I was always amazed that he could hold his arm out that long with no support.

After the drain was complete, Bill replenished with good energy Pete's same energy fields that had been drained. Pete's energy fields would change, returning once again to a high-frequency level. There were times when Bill's arms and hands shook uncontrollably with the force of the energy coursing through his body and back into Pete's. Once replenished, Bill would laugh and tell Pete, "God sure loves you, Pete. You have a beautiful soul." Bill would exclaim this while shaking out his arms and hands, much like an athlete would do after running a long race.

Other times, Bill assessed that Pete's energy fields needed to be aligned. The energy fields surrounding Pete's body, called an aura, were off-center to either side, or crawled up Pete's body so it was not centered. This re-alignment increased Pete's energy flows, too.

Bill did many different kinds of healing treatments over the months he worked on Pete. Sometimes he was led to use light on an energy field. He was always led to a specific color of light, such as green or gold. Bill would use energy of that color to then do his work. At the end of each session Bill would ask God if any other work was needed to be done. If the answer was "No," the session would end.

The swelling in Pete's legs and ankles was visibly down after Bill did Healing Touch for his blood clots. Pete's resilience during his radiation could be explained by the power of Bill's work in cleansing Pete's energy fields from the toxins caused by the radiation. Bill never claimed to do any healing himself. "I am just the instrument," he'd say. We could never prove that Healing Touch was responsible for any specific healing of Pete. Pete and I both agreed that it surely didn't do any harm.

The archangels were with Pete frequently when Bill came to do his work. I never saw the angels, but Bill would feel their presence by the intensity of energy around Pete. I remember one day when Bill opened the door and walked into our living room. Pete was sitting in his chair, which was about fifteen feet from our front door. Pete looked up and gave Bill one of those warm, welcoming smiles that Pete always gave Bill when he saw him. Bill stopped dead in his tracks inside the door. He grinned.

"We have company today!" Bill exclaimed. He put out his hands like he was feeling a big bubble. "I can feel the energy from here."

"Oh yeah," I said. "Who's here?"

"Well, let me see," Bill said. He closed his eyes and asked for guidance. "The archangels are here," he said with excitement in his voice. "All four of them, Pete! You must be pretty special!"

Bill said the amount of energy in the room was amazing. The angels stayed for the whole Healing Touch session. Bill knew when they left. I was overwhelmed with feelings of reverence. The three of us prayed in thanksgiving together.

There was one instance when Bill gave me two instructions that he said he got when working on Pete. He told me he was directed to tell me to: "Get another MRI done now and then stop radiation."

I really believed Bill was a messenger from God for Pete. I had obeyed other instructions sent to me through Bill. But in this instance, I felt so conflicted about stopping radiation. It did not feel right to me. I prayed over it. I asked God to give me guidance. I finally asked Nan what she thought, and she said to dismiss Bill's instruction.

She told me, "I got after him after he made that comment to you. To put Kathy in that position is untenable. Don't do it again."

I felt relief. I understood now how much of a healing team they were. Bill did not operate independently. And neither did God. I felt peace.

On a daily basis, I assisted Bill's healing of Pete by doing Healing Touch on Pete through a simple energy field clearing technique Bill had taught me. I'd put my two hands together over Pete's head while he was sitting in his favorite chair. He'd turn off the TV, close his eyes and relax. I'd then sweep down over Pete's body with a conscious intention to clear any toxins that may have settled in Pete's energy fields that day. I did about thirty-five sweeps, praying as I did them. Pete would pray, too. I dusted my hands away from Pete's body after each sweep. I'd finish by fanning the bottom of each of his feet twenty-five times, since toxins tended to settle in the lowest point of his body. We rarely missed a day. After I finished, Pete would open his eyes and tell me thank you with the most loving of looks. It was always a very peaceful and intimate moment for us.

Pete and I received many suggestions from friends and business associates for alternative healing treatment options during Pete's journey. It was overwhelming to me and to Pete to try to figure out which ones we should research or pursue. Neither of us had the energy or the time to sort out all these options. Bill knew about many alternative treatments. Bill's love for Pete was without question. He would screen for us all non-traditional healing suggestions. He'd research any options he was not familiar with. Bill paid us a real service by screening others' ideas. We trusted him completely.

At Bill's suggestion, Pete and I visited a doctor who was a medical intuitor. Bill and Nan went with us. Many experienced nurses said they "trusted this doctor's assessments more than MRI results." This doctor healed by sight, while Bill healed by touch. She told us that she could see different vibration rates of energy fields. She assessed Pete by having him sit in a chair in front of her.

"Diseases have different energy vibration rates and colors," she explained. "Cancer has a very low vibration rate, and is black in color in the energy fields. I don't sense anything critical in you, Pete. I don't sense that you are dying. I don't see any areas of black which would be cancer."

She did find that energy was leaking from Pete's head and so she plugged the holes in his head, energetically speaking. She was a lot more concerned about Pete's digestive system.

"It's weak," she told Pete. "You are not absorbing as much nutrition as you should from the food you are eating." She advised us to switch to organic foods, stop microwaving foods since it destroyed much of the nutrients, and not eat fast foods. Bill then worked with the doctor on Pete's digestive system. The doctor gave Bill some advice as to what kind of healing treatments he should use with Pete.

I was ecstatic that this doctor had found no cancer, and that Pete's death was not imminent from her perspective. I felt relief. Pete treated the visit matter-of-factly. He was more concerned about the lack of feeling in his right arm and leg. The doctor didn't think that his lack of sensation had anything to do with his brain cancer. She referred us to a chiropractor. We did follow-up with the chiropractor, and he disagreed with the medical intuitor. He thought it had everything to do with Pete's brain tumor. He told us he couldn't do anything for Pete. We appreciated his honesty, and lost a little enthusiasm for the medical intuitor. But Pete and I did make a change in our grocery shopping habits. We changed to a store that carried more organic foods, and made as many organic food purchases as possible.

From my prayer journal: March of 2006

Bill and I witnessed your power and your energy flowing into Pete again yesterday. All the archangels were here—Michael, Raphael, Gabriel and Uriel. The Holy Spirit was present. Thank you for your presence. I don't know what result you are creating. Are you readying Pete to take him to another place? Are you here to heal and restore him? I believe in your power. I witnessed you yesterday. Whatever the result, may it be your glory, Lord! Where you lead, I will follow.

13

A New Normal

By May of 2006, Pete moved to a new normal. On the medical front, Pete successfully transitioned from Depakote to Topamax, both anti-seizure medications, which Dr. Albright believed would help his platelet count rebound. In fact it did, reaching a count of one hundred and thirty-two thousand. WOW! Pete gained another two pounds, and Dr. Albright exclaimed that "everything is better." Pete's blood counts were getting close to the normal range. All aspects of Pete's nutrition profile improved.

Dr. Albright pulled his computer screen into the examination room on a portable cart. Pete and I waited as he searched the screens to find the right version of Pete's latest MRI. The waiting felt like forever. It was totally silent in the room.

I had asked Pete the night before if he was nervous about getting the results of the MRI.

"The answer is the answer," he said. "And I am doing better and getting closer to normal and that gives me hope."

We all sat and watched the picture of Pete's brain on the screen.

"No sign of a tumor and no sign of any tumor activity!" Dr. Albright exclaimed. "A dramatic change for the better." And that's the closest our doctor ever got to enthusiasm. Dr. Albright went on. "Well, since this looks so good you have some options now, Pete. You can do nothing other than monitor the situation every thirty days with a new MRI. Or you could finally start taking Temodar, since your platelet counts have finally gotten normal." Temodar was an oral chemotherapy agent which would have normally been given as a standard treatment with the radiation Pete had finished.

Pete opted for no new treatment. I agreed. Pete's only question was "Will I ever be able to drive a car again?"

Dr. Albright didn't say no. "Your occupational therapist can help you get ready to re-take a driver's test, and if you pass the test, Pete, I'll sign off on the order to okay you to drive."

Pete's face lit up. I let out a "whoo-hoo." Before we left the doctor's office Pete and I joined hands with Mary Jo, bowed our heads and thanked God for His work. It felt like a miracle to me!

Pete's Carepage: May 4, 2006 @ 9:31 p.m.

"Dramatically improved," the doc said. "Unusual to see this type of tumor have this kind of result. No evidence of any tumor-like activity," Dr A said. Feels like a miracle to me and Pete! Make a BIG deal of God's awesome work and his warrior archangels—Michael, Uriel, and Raphael. Our hearts are full of gratitude and our eyes have tears of joy! Awesome God. Pete cannot express—I cannot express—the happiness we feel and the thankfulness and appreciation we feel for God and all of you. Your prayers have lifted us. Your love sustained us. Your hearts have given us comfort, in addition to all the meals, ice cream, and goodies of all sorts, and cards, and gifts and books. We can't thank you enough. Join us in choruses of praise for God's love and mercy. You have all been amazing!

§ § § § §

One Response to Pete's Carepage: Answered Prayers

Several weeks ago, I mentioned to a friend that I was having difficulty keeping track of all the people that I wanted to pray for, as my list seemed to grow by the day over the past few months (including the two of you). It was suggested that I only create a prayer book, but that I also include the date that God had answered each prayer so that I reflect back (when life gets tough) and give Him praise and thanks for answered prayers.

I am so, so excited to be able to put May 4th next to your names. That doesn't mean that you won't be in my prayers and thoughts—you will.

I am so amazed with the faith that the two of you
have demonstrated during this difficult time.
You've been such strong disciples during the tough-
est of situations and have let the love of Christ
shine through you to others! That deserves a big
"whoo hoo!"

Sherri

Before we left the doctor's office, we asked to have Pete's PICC
line removed. The doctor agreed, which meant he didn't expect to
need it for chemotherapy or blood tests or IVs. For the first time in
months, Pete had his left arm back, and didn't have to worry about
that old PICC line dangling out from the sleeve of his shirts. I didn't
have to cleanse it with saline and heparin syringes daily. Now we had
no need for a visiting nurse, since her primary reason for visiting was
to monitor Pete's PICC line. Small things to celebrate! It felt good to
throw out all those syringes and supplies! Could our life be getting
back to a new normal?

Shortly thereafter, we had a conference with our three therapists:
physical, occupational and speech. They all gave approval for Pete's
independence. No more need for twenty-four-hour supervision.
Another "whoo-hoo!" We agreed to set up a plan for emergencies if
Pete would ever need to call 911. All three therapists agreed that Pete
could get out of the house on his own if his safety was threatened.
Another milestone!

On the personal front, Pete returned to a new normal, too. He
started to answer the phone again when it rang, and he'd get the message right. In his professional life, Pete had probably spent almost
eight hours a day on the phone every day for the last fifteen years. It
was as comfortable to him as breathing. He started initiating calls on
his own, looking up numbers in his address book without a problem.
I'd overhear his conversations. They were short, but clear.

Pete started going downstairs to our bedroom, managing all sixteen
steps without a cane, at first just for naps, but by June we had moved
back full time into our own bedroom and master bath. Signs of recovery!

Pete swept the garage, a chore he had a passion for doing, since I
didn't seem to be bothered by the leaves blown into the corners of the
garage. He swept our deck, which was his second most favorite chore
after the garage. After he swept the deck, he fired up his beloved
smoker. He had no problems remembering how to use it. He made

"Pete's Best Ribs" with no help from me, and we savored every morsel. While the ribs were smoking, which takes a few hours, Pete and I laid down in our two-person hammock, which was on our deck right next to the smoker. He turned his head and smiled at me. "I'm really happy," he said genuinely. I treasured that moment; it was precious to me.

We went to my Mom and Dad's for a family celebration, and Pete walked in with a cane, but under his own power. He wanted no assistance! Pete shared with me how embarrassed he was that he couldn't remember names. "Not even the family," he said, looking at me in agony.

"Who cares about names?" I'd say sincerely. "Everyone understands."

Pete was such a courteous person. He would never offend someone knowingly, and he hated to be embarrassed in front of others. Finally, he just stopped using names completely. Even mine.

Pete made it to a Red's ballgame. Pete loved baseball. He would watch every Cincinnati Reds televised game starting with spring training. Sitting in his chair, watching the ballgame with his feet propped up on his footstool, sent a clear message that "all is right with the world." Pete was happy and at peace. Getting to the ballgame was a special treat. We took my dad, another avid baseball fan, with us, as well as Mike, Mary Jo and Mom. Even though Pete wasn't using a wheelchair anymore, Mike had asked for handicapped seating when buying the tickets a few weeks prior. So Pete agreed to go in the wheelchair, and as a result we got the best seats in the house! The Reds beat the St Louis Cardinals that day, 3–2 in the bottom of the ninth to go up two games in the division, and post the best record so far in baseball. Oh my. In recent years, the Reds were constant cellar dwellers in baseball. I took it as a good omen—miracles do happen!

Mary Jo and Mike helped us make special memories by going with us to Cincinnati's five-star restaurant to celebrate our twenty-first wedding anniversary. The menu was individualized with the headline, "Happy 21st Anniversary Pete & Kathy." The chef himself came out to autograph it. Pete was so pleased. It delighted him to have a person of influence, be it a chef, a pastor, or our bank CEO, take special notice of him or me. On this night, Pete had his first class of wine since surgery!

Pete was a member of a CEO Roundtable group sponsored by the Cincinnati Chamber of Commerce. He had been a member of the group for the last ten years or so. They met at seven-thirty a.m. at a

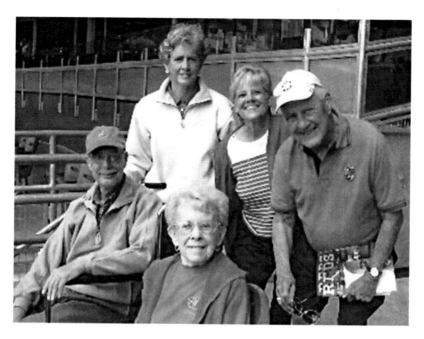

Pete, Kathy, Mary Jo, Mom, and Dad at the Reds Game

member's place of business. He hadn't attended a meeting since December. Pete got himself up at six-thirty to make the May CEO Roundtable meeting. I drove him and walked with him into the meeting. What a look of delight on his colleagues' faces! They got up and began greeting him all at once, words tumbling out in rapid fire. Pete just grinned, shaking hands all around and steadying himself with a chair. Then he grinned some more. Happiness filled that conference room that day. A rather low-key group, joyous in reuniting.

When Pete came home he said he really enjoyed the meeting. I asked him what was discussed. He said they always ran their meetings the same way. Each person gave themselves two rankings, one for personal and one for professional, reflecting their level of satisfaction on a scale of one to ten. Then they would talk about the basis for their rankings.

"I gave myself an eight for personal happiness. For work, I gave a one and a nine. A one because I am not working; a nine because I am so happy."

How he lifted my heart through those words! I grinned at him and gave him a kiss.

Next, Pete invited the Angus group, his company, over to our house for a Montgomery Inn rib dinner. He greeted each person as they came in. More hugs from this group! Lots of chatter. Excitement. It was electric in our dining room. The stories they told of clients and the inquiries about him from them. The almost-closed cases brought sighs. They bragged on their successes. They assured Pete that his tradition of honking the horn when a placement was made was being carried on faithfully. The look on his face as they made a toast to his recovery was a sight to behold. He'd say his eyes misted over.

Everyone confirmed that Pete was doing well. I was struck by the fact that Pete's healing came through relationships, lots of them: the medical team, the therapy team, the Crossroads team, our friends and business associates joined in a community through Carepages, our family, and Healing Touch. Healing didn't come in isolation. And it was about at this moment that Bill announced he would stop coming daily to do healing touch on Pete.

"Pete is getting better," Bill said. "He doesn't need me every day anymore. I'll start coming on a weekly basis, just to monitor."

I was afraid to believe that God was in fact healing Pete. Too good to be true!

Pete and I started a routine of daily walking. Pete hated doing his physical therapy exercises so much that walking was a good substitute for him and for me. It kept me from having to push him to exercise, and walking was something we both loved. There was a park below our house that was international in design, capturing and sorting plants from all over the world. How I loved walking amid the tall grasses of Africa, or in an English garden! Pete made eight hundred steps the first day. He wanted me to count his steps. Each day a little further, a few more steps. He was driven! He responded well to the challenge.

Pete taught me patience. He taught me the value of slowing down and enjoying the moment. When we walked each day, I noticed the day. I noticed the hour of the day, where the sun was in the sky and how the shadows played. As Pete got stronger we were able to make it to the end of the park, which was about a half-mile out and a half-mile back. A construction site of town homes across the street from the park where we walked captured Pete's attention. How he loved to stop and watch the workers! All summer we watched. It was a fun game. Each time we walked, we competed with each other to see who noticed the most changes since the last walk. The town homes progressed, just like he progressed. The retaining wall was done! The pouring of the foundation took days and days, the big concrete trucks lumbering up and down the street with their constant hum. Finally the lumber was going up, and then the roof. I'd watch Pete's face as he watched. He was engrossed, with such a peaceful and pleasant look on his face. He rarely ever said a word.

Pete had taken out a long-term disability insurance policy after he bought his own business in 1997, to partially protect his income in case anything ever happened to him. How smart that decision now seemed to be! Making a claim for that insurance was easy. Pete started receiving payments right away. All that was required was certification of his medical diagnosis, and periodic follow-up reports from the doctor. Since he paid for this insurance himself, none of this income was taxable.

We also knew Pete would be eligible for disability benefits from Social Security. Accessing those funds was a lot more difficult. Pete and I sat at the computer, filling out page after page of the application. The application timed out on the computer as we looked for something requested, and we had a hard time retrieving what we had already submitted. It took us hours to fill out the application, only to find out that the Social Security administration would not accept an online application since the application was for disability benefits, and Pete wasn't sixty-two. Those parameters kicked us out of the online process.

I was so frustrated! I called the local Social Security office and made an appointment. I remember Pete and me sitting in this big cafeteria-style room waiting for our number to be called. The Social Security staff sat in teller-like windows and looked out at all of us poor people waiting. Actually, once we saw someone in person, the process flew. She reached out with kindness to help us, and facilitated our application which had, in fact, been captured and stored online, so we didn't have to repeat that whole process! Pete was eligible for benefits from six months after diagnosis. We received a Social Security payment at the end of October for July 2006 (first month of Pete's eligibility) and for every month thereafter. Pete was delighted. He felt good about getting some benefit for all those years his earnings had been taxed!

How amazing Pete was in terms of his level of activity. There were still very tired days when Pete would sleep a lot of the day away. But those days became the exception. Pete loved going out to dinner, so we started going out to dinners regularly with friends: the Knotty Pine for Bayou food with our boating friends; the Golden Lamb, an old historic inn in Lebanon Ohio with friends Bill and Nan and Robin. Pete grilled lamb chops for dinner at home.

We visited both the eye doctor and the ear doctor at Pete's request. He felt his vision and hearing was still a problem. And they were. Not major obstacles, but he had definite diminishment in his hearing probably due to the radiation. His long-distance vision had improved, although he periodically experienced double vision at a distance. Pete compensated well so it was not giving him major problems, and the eye doctor thought it might go away with time. Another side effect from the radiation, probably. But his short distance reading had gotten worse, so the doctor made a slight adjustment to Pete's prescription.

I was being honored at a United Way event in early May that year. I was the recipient of the New Century Leadership Award for the work I had done in co-founding the Women's Leadership Council in the Greater Cincinnati United Way. Pete wanted to come. How much his presence meant to me, because I knew all too well the cost to him in terms of effort.

This was a large luncheon event at the city's convention center. The halls were massive. The luncheon was in the third-floor ballroom, which meant Pete had to come up two long and steep escalators. To get to those escalators he had to walk down a long hall, since the escalators and the ballroom were at the very opposite side of the closest handicapped entrance.

I had to get to the ballroom early for pictures and a rehearsal. I couldn't take Pete to the event. Mary Jo and Mike and other family members volunteered to take Pete there. When I finished the rehearsal, I stood out in the center of the hall looking through the crowds for Pete.

Then I saw him. I smiled. My eyes filled with tears. There he was slowly walking down that long convention center hall. He had refused to use a wheelchair. "No cart," he told my sister emphatically. So there he was in a sports coat and tie, with his ball cap covering the surgery scar on his head, step by slow step getting closer to me. He saw me. I waved.

Pete stood next to me in the lobby of the meeting hall with a grin on his face a mile wide, beaming with a pride that said "this is my wife and she is getting honored today." People came streaming up to see Pete and shake his hand. He was the real guest of honor! Everyone knew Pete in the city, and hadn't seen him since his surgery. I was the proud one, standing next to him watching him smile and shake hands. I felt his tension as he strained to remember names. But it didn't matter. He had a blast. It was Pete's coming out! Amidst the hundreds of people there, he wore the only hat in the place!

Pete's Carepage: May 12, 2006 @ 5:50 p.m.

This is Pete. I send a quick note about the latest physical results for me. This week the doctors were able to determine that the blood clots in my legs are no longer there! Hurray! Added to the wonderful news from the MRI last week that for the moment the cancer is gone and there is no sign of a tumor. I have been pretty happy all week! How much I appreciate all the notes, messages, prayers and gifts you have all sent me.

This is Kathy. For all you who were praying for the blood clots to dissolve—they have! The technician kept looking, expecting to find them, but they were not there! We were all surprised that they would have dissolved so soon. The doc reminded us that there is a fifty percent chance of recurrence of the clots—but for now we can stop the treatment. No more shots of blood thinner in Pete's stomach. More thanks to God and all of you faithful pray-ers!

This Sunday at our church, Crossroads will gather us to join in a prayer of thanksgiving and praise to God for all the good works He has done for Pete and through Pete! Know that each and every one of you will be in my heart as I give Thanksgiving. So if you feel a "bolt of energy" around 10:00 a.m. Sunday—know that is coming from us! I am so aware of the many "communities" made up of each of you and all of you that have been the "Lift" beneath our wings. We will never be able to thank you enough. Pete and I are humbled before your generous outpouring of love and support.

§ § § § §

One Carepage response: Emma

While at Valida and Bruce's to see the new baby girl Sally August, I saw and felt something marvelous. Emma was saying grace at dinner. Her version is the "Now I lay me down to sleep." At only 3 yrs old that has meaning to her. At the end with the God Blesses she added and 'God Bless Pete." Then she announced "OK Eat." What a wonder

Yes I will join you in heart and mind when you celebrate and thank everyone at Crossroads on Sunday. I am sure I will feel the "jolt." Continue the

```
good fight and we will soon all be together looking
back on the challenge you both met head on.
```

```
Judith
```

That evening we went out to dinner with our neighbors Cheryl and Amit. Cheryl, who was a breast cancer survivor, asked Pete, "Are you afraid? Living with all the uncertainty?"

Pete said, "I don't feel fear. Whatever God's plan is, I accept."

Pete showed such peace. Each morning we would pray before breakfast. Most days this was Pete's prayer. "I thank you, God, for waking up again this morning. Thanks for another great day. Amen."

My father went into the hospital on May 18 for a bowel re-section. His doctors had discovered that Dad had colon cancer.

He looked at my mother with sadness. "After all these years and cancer is finally going to get me."

My father was eighty-four years old, and a healthy eighty-four-year old. His recovery from the colon surgery was slow and complicated by heart issues and then pneumonia. He was in the hospital for thirty-eight days.

For each of those days, Pete and I visited him. I couldn't believe Pete's willingness and determination to see my dad every day. Those visits to my father in the hospital were in addition to Pete's multiple therapy visits at Good Samaritan Hospital. Pete never flinched. I told him we could skip a day. I told him multiple times he didn't have to go today.

He'd say, "I'll just make a short stop in to see Dad." He always went. He taught me some things through those hospital visits. He taught me about faithfulness. The importance of just being there. He taught me about loyalty. He would say just a few short words to Dad, usually about the Reds or the weather. Together, he and my dad would look out the window in Dad's hospital room and count the number of yellow cars in the parking lot. It was their game. With Pete's word-finding problems and my dad's hearing problems, they could only communicate in a type of quiet man-to-man speak. Pete would put his thumbs up to give my dad encouragement, and my dad would light up when he saw Pete come into the room. The love between them was palpable.

Pete's Carepage: June 8, 2006 @ 10:43 p.m.

I have received a few calls over the last week asking how Pete was doing since I haven't been posting updates anymore! I feel so lucky that there are so many of you STILL have such an interest in support-ing us. How lucky we are!

No updates mean no significant news! And I guess that IS signifi-cant news! Pete is doing very well. He gets stronger every day. We still go to the hospital two days every week for three therapy sessions each of those days. He walks now without assistance always. The wheelchair is in mothballs until someone else in the family/friends needs it. YEAH! Our physical therapist is starting to talk about his work with Pete nearing completion. We got the boat in the water—YEAH! Even though it hasn't left the dock. Pete can walk to the slip, handling the "moving dock and boat just fine." In occupational ther-apy, Pete's goal is to be able to drive again. We did a formal assess-ment today to get him to an actual driving instructor that would certify his readiness to drive to the doctor. The only real obstacle is Pete's reaction times are still slow, but we will keep at it. Speech and memory lags the physical improvements. His word-finding is much better but reading comprehension is still weak. I taped our address and phone number on our phone so Pete could remember.

But life is good. We treasure every day as special. The slowness of our life now has a totally different and wonderful sense of joy. As many of you told me, and encouraged me to discover. And it is so. We give thanks to God many times each day and continue to give Him the glory for both of our healing. I've told Pete his physical healing was God's miracle in him and the "spirit healing" God has given me through Pete is miraculous, too. His love for both of us continues to be shown over and over again in all of you. I will never be able to express the gratitude I have for each and all of you.

PS The Cleveland Clinic finally reviewed Pete's MRI of May 4 with their Tumor Board. I trust the expertise so much of Dr B (our sur-geon) and his staff at the clinic. They said that Pete's MRI couldn't have looked any better. They were amazed! (And taking credit for the IL-13 treatment which is just fine!) No further treatment is recom-mended by them-just MRI's every eight weeks to make sure nothing recurs. Our next MRI will be the first week in July. Praise God!

The occupational therapist had cleared Pete to take his driving test. The day before his test we went up to my old high school, the place my dad had taught me to drive. Pete drove the car for the first time since his surgeries. We practiced in the parking lot. Turns and stops. Did parallel parking. He had absolutely no problems at all. His confi-dence grew. We decided to leave the safe haven of my high school parking lot, and head to the expressway. We ran an errand for my father, which required about twelve miles of expressway driving. Pete performed like an ace.

Pete's Carepage: June 21,206 @ 11:53am

More GOOD NEWS! I passed the driving test today! I had the opportunity to undertake the driving exam for getting the "no driving" restriction eliminated. I have had this restriction since surgery back in January and have been working with our occupational therapist to get ready for the test today. I am so happy! Kathy and I will now be able to share the driving during our trip to Florida to see son Mike and family/friends along the way in our new station wagon next week.

§ § § § §

Response to Pete's Carepage: You are an Inspiration

```
Pete—congrats on the driving test. You are an
inspiration to us all. May God continue to bless
you and Kathy.
```

Todd

That same week, Pete graduated from physical therapy too, passing the balance test with an equilibrium score of seventy-four vs. a norm of sixty-nine. Pete was beaming. On July 6, Pete had his next MRI. Dr. Albright said Pete's MRI looked clean! "The healing continues," I thought with relief. Dr. Albright's recommendation was just to monitor every eight weeks through an MRI.

That recommendation changed by the time I got the clinic's assessment. They said they could see a small enhancement (which is brain doctorese for bad stuff when they don't know what it is) at the base of Pete's brain. They said it could be medication because the new enhancement was at one of the IL-13 catheter sites. My heart froze in fear.

They continued, "We don't want to do anything different right now, let's just move the next MRI and review in thirty days instead of sixty days."

I breathed easier. We could do that. And so we did. For the next year, Pete would get an MRI every thirty days followed by a visit with Dr. Albright and a review by the Cleveland Clinic. We asked Bill about the enhancement. The message he got was that it was just the drug.

We asked Mary Jo to leave the examination room during the visit with Dr. Albright so Pete could ask Dr. Albright about the impact of his brain tumor on his sexuality. Pete was so intent. He really wanted an answer!

Dr. Albright really didn't answer Pete. He tested his testosterone level, thinking that the radiation and medication may have gotten Pete's hormones out of balance. Pete's testosterone level tested normal. We asked him if Pete's surgery could have affected the sexual center in Pete's brain. Dr. Albright said sexuality is not located anywhere specific in the brain, and it is located everywhere in the brain. Dr. Albright told us that no one really knew where sexuality was located in the brain. So it is not anywhere, but it is everywhere. What were we supposed to do with that? Pete just wanted to know what he could do about it! No one had told us of this side-effect of brain surgery. Pete was frustrated and disappointed.

I started researching everything I could find on sexual function post brain surgery. I couldn't find anything in the medical guides other than some advice about enjoying "intimacy in new ways." Hmm. Pete and I realized we were on our own in this arena. There were no good answers.

Pete was the most sexual man I had ever known. He and I had a healthy sexual relationship. We made love often, and it was very satisfying for both of us. The trust between us was unshakable. Pete was intent on continuing the sexual aspect of our relationship. And he did. Even when his medications and physical symptoms inhibited his enjoyment, he persisted in making me happy. We both enjoyed the intimacy even when we had physical limitations. One day while we were in bed, he thanked me for not cheating on him while he was sick. I was curled up in his arms. I looked up at him and cried tears of astonishment that he would even worry about this. And then I cried tears for his generosity.

In all other areas, Pete was getting better. All we had left was speech therapy. Pete hated speech therapy. He'd get so frustrated when he couldn't name simple things correctly. Our speech therapist gave us a software program we could use at home to do exercises, and Pete would do them, but all the while gritting his teeth. His speech improved dramatically in the month of July. His word-finding was much better, and his sentence structure kept getting more complex. He was writing on his own and reading more. One day he sat at his chair and wrote his first letter. It was to his college roommate Steelman. It was two pages and it took him over two hours. Pete graduated from speech therapy in August! All the therapies were now finished! Huge milestone for us.

From my prayer journal: July of 2006

Praise to you, Lord. Pete is recovering more and more. Nan and Bill saw him after three weeks away today and how much better he seemed to them. His word-finding. His sentence structure getting more complex. Thank you! Thank you!

Show me the way to be his own personal angel. To help him stay active and alert. He is a fighter. He faces challenges every day. He must get so discouraged. He's motivated by trips. Help me understand what gives him satisfaction now. Not in the old days. But now.

Pete gives me lots of pleasure. He is more direct now with his feelings and desires. He laughs more now. And we have wonderful days of appreciating the small things together. I give thanks. I remember—You are the Path. I have no idea where this journey will lead us. Possibly more nightmares. Possibly more challenges. Possibly Pete losing more capacity. But I know you will not leave us. You are faithful. You will not abandon Pete—or me. We trust in you.

14

My New Normal

My life had changed dramatically, from a busy executive who triple-booked events and traveled constantly, to a caregiver of Pete's. Our friends sympathized with Pete, knowing he was now the sole focus of my unbounded energy! But he wasn't complaining, and neither was I. The only things that didn't change for me was my prayer routine in the early morning before Pete awoke, and my exercise routine of running at least three times a week. Other than that, I didn't recognize the life I was leading. My time and energy were now spent on researching brain tumors and their treatment; managing doctors' appointments and therapy routines; caring for the household tasks and caring for Pete. That meant cooking and laundry and paying bills and home maintenance. I resigned from two volunteer boards I was on and kept volunteer board assignments with two others. I always weighed time away from Pete seriously, and only went to things I needed to attend. I eliminated any discretionary activities.

By May of 2006, I needed to resolve my employment situation with the bank. The bank had given me an open-ended leave of absence, and I did not want to abuse their generosity. I hadn't worked since January 13, 2006, and summer was fast approaching. They had not replaced me yet. Chuck, one of the managers who worked for me, had taken on the majority of my responsibilities in addition to his own. That was not fair to him.

I knew I did not want to go back to the bank. Others at the bank, as well as family and friends, could not imagine that I didn't want to return. I had been so engaged and so happy there. US Bank had been so much of my life. All true. But for me, this was not an agonizing decision. In fact, I couldn't remember any previous career decision that had been as certain as this one was for me.

The bank's generosity to Pete and me during the twenty-two years I had worked there made my working not a financial decision for us. The bank allowed my health benefits to continue, which was a huge consideration, since Pete was covered under my health benefits. How humbled and full of thanks I was. All I could feel was gratefulness. Clearly I had worked hard for the bank, but many others had worked hard for their employers too, and were not treated as well as I was being treated. I saw God's abundance in the bank's generosity toward Pete and me.

So the decision to return or not to return to work had to do with where I wanted to focus my energies and attention. I had always had a chronic, gnawing, underlying question about my purpose in life. I had answered that question peacefully many times before, but now I had a new answer and it came like a neon sign—a flashing neon sign!

Never before had it been so clear. I think that is why I felt such certainty. It came immediately. "This changes everything," I had said to Pete when he told me the radiologists thought he had a brain tumor. My response was not from me. And from that minute, in those brief and truthful seconds passing between us, glance to glance, in the painful tear-filled looks exchanged, I understood what it meant to have a clear communication from the almighty. I knew now what my purpose was. And I was going to be obedient. In serving Pete, I fulfilled my mission: to love and serve Pete with everything I had, and to do so with excellence. Pete deserved excellence.

And in that decision, I felt a freedom and a joy I had never before experienced. It was exhilarating.

I had heard God speaking to me before, but never in such a loud and clear way. I knew that in making the care of Pete my sole focus, I was submitting to Pete and obeying God. My old life slipped away. I felt God's presence in me, and between Pete and me. I felt an overflowing love for Pete. It was not a hard decision. It was not an effort. I didn't worry about losing my career. It didn't matter anymore. No more driving hard for results, or fulfilling my career ambitions. It was the easiest decision that I had ever made.

My life became all about listening to Pete, and paying attention to every detail about Pete. In doing that I was slowly transformed, not just with Pete but with others, too. I surprised myself: I was really listening to someone, not just pretending that I was. I appreciated others more. "Thanks" became a frequent expression of mine. I became less focused on tasks. I became less critical, less judgmental. Driving hard for the next thing was not as important as holding dear the moment that was. It was the love between Pete and me that was important.

I had a new mission. I knew I'd miss my banking team, but realized even though the team was lost, the individuals were not. Some would now become friends. And those relationships would withstand the change, because they were based on love. Whenever fears about my future did surface, I'd re-focus on my love for Pete and my fears would be chased away.

I called my boss Richard, who was also my friend, on May 26 and told him I would not be returning to my current position at the bank on July 1, a date we had agreed to.

"Well, July is arbitrary, Kathy," Richard said. "Could you be back by August or September? We have waited this long; we can wait a little longer."

It was clear Richard wanted me to come back. I also knew he understood. "Pete's not ready for my return," I said.

"If that's the only reason you have for not returning, I can accept that. I kept avoiding calling you," Richard said," because I didn't want to have this conversation."

"I know. Me either. But I wanted to give you as much notice as possible."

"Ours is a life-long relationship," he said. "No one has been as close to me in all that I've been through as you. And that is really all that matters. And you know you have a job at the bank whenever and wherever you want it."

I was silent as I hung up. So much had changed for me. My heart had changed. I didn't have the enthusiasm for the work or the bank like I had before. I wanted to honor the bank. I loved the bank. And I was so grateful. But I didn't want to go back to my old world. This decision was really just a logical extension of my decision made months ago about obeying God by serving Pete.

I held a conference call with all the managers who reported directly to me, as well as all the partners who supported our business. I offered to have one-on-one conversations with whoever wanted one. There was lots of silence on the phone that day. They said they weren't surprised. They talked about how much they missed my personal touch and my care for them as individuals. They respected and understood my decision. They kindly shared with me the positive impact I had had on them.

As I hung up, I felt freed to love them as people now—not as a useful resource to the company. And I felt a loss. I felt a loss of a whole life. I knew my work would get dismantled by whoever replaced me. And in that moment I saw, in a philosophical way, the futility of all work and of all tasks. The only thing that really lasted was who we have become though the work we have done and the people we have loved in doing that work. It is how that love has changed us that matters most and remains.

A few months prior to my announcement, I had the chance to do a video message for the bank's annual recognition ceremony, "The Pinnacle." It was the biggest event of the year for my team and all the members of their teams. Held in a resort kind of environment, the bank recognized the top ten percent of district, branch and sales managers and their spouses or significant others. There would usually be about a thousand people attending an event like this. It was a black-tie affair with fireworks, giveaways and lots of entertainment. I had always given a keynote type of speech at these events in the past, and was invited to do so again, even though I could not be physically present. I used this event to share with my team what I had learned so far in my journey with Pete.

I told them how lucky I felt to have this chance to care for Pete. To pay him back for all the years he had supported me at the bank. I told them how generous the bank had been to me, to give me this chance. And I told them, "Love is the only thing that matters. It is the one thing that is eternal."

The bank sent me a video of the event, and as the camera scanned the crowds, hundreds of faces I knew were captured on the screen. Some were crying. Some were smiling and waving. I could read their lips. "Kathy, we love you, too." Pete and I watched with tears in our eyes. Although I hadn't realized it at the time, it was the right way to say good-bye.

What I missed the most about leaving the bank was the corporate identity that working in a large company gave me. I didn't know how to answer the question, "What do you do?" I used to say that I was a banker. Or that I worked for US Bank. I wondered if God could give me a good new answer to that question. Would he give me something of his to replace my old corporate identity and the perquisites that went with it?

I had just lost so many advantages that I had taken for granted for so long. Talk about going into a zone where I wasn't comfortable! I had been taken care of by two assistants for the last several years. Now I lost assistants, my cell phone, my computer, my Blackberry, and all the resources of a large corporation in one fell swoop. I hadn't even made an airline reservation for myself in years. How spoiled I was! I was embarrassed. I had to learn everything new.

Mike helped me get a new laptop. He set up the software for me. Then I started humbly and patiently learning how to do simple things that others had done for me for so many years: building file folders, cutting and pasting, building an address book. Making my own travel plans. Corporate advantages gone! And my identity, too?

I cleaned out my desk July 28. Both of my assistants came in one evening to help me. We shared an intimacy from years of working together. They were special to me. I was special to them. We drank a cold beer as we emptied files into the dumpsters. I felt like I had just had a divorce.

Pete and I both thanked God for releasing us from the burden of work. I was not unhappy at all. I even surprised myself when I completed a lifeline exercise as part of our small group, all-church journey at Crossroads. We were tasked with doing a lifeline marking our high and low points from a midline spanning our life from kindergarten years to current. I expected to have Pete's diagnosis as one of my low points on the lifeline, but in fact, as I captured my feelings and identified real low points in my life, Pete's diagnosis and the change that resulted for me was not a low point at all. In fact, at only one other time in my life had I felt as good, and was the line as high from the midline as it was now.

The overall sense of happiness, however, did not eliminate some very painful moments. It was only after Pete recovered that I realized he would never be the same Pete as he was before his surgeries. I think I knew this intellectually, but as he got better I realized it. I had lost some of Pete already. Pete would never be the same Pete. I felt resentful about the tasks I now needed to do that he had always done: taking out the garbage, paying the bills and driving all the financial decisions for us. Pete had always done all those. He had taken care of most of the issues around the house—now they were mine to worry about and do. I felt a strong sense of loss. And with the realization of the loss, a heavy sadness seeped in.

What was a blessing to both of us was that Pete still understood everything. He and I had conversations about every one of those items he used to do. He just didn't think about them on his own. I had to bring them up. He didn't take ownership anymore, but we could discuss anything I wanted to raise. The brilliant firepower of his brain was still there. He'd be able to direct me to where things were that I couldn't find, and he had strong opinions on most issues. I don't think I can remember one decision affecting our life that he wasn't party to. Most of the time, I followed his lead. He would delight in our conversations. He loved to show me where he had put things. It was like he was preparing me for the time when he'd be gone. I didn't want to be prepared! But things had changed. I now had the responsibility and he was the helper.

From my prayer journal: April of 2006

Thank you for sunrises. We know not what we shall become. Uncertainty and certainty. Certainty about you. Your presence. Your love. Pleasing you by obeying your commands. Everything else is uncertain. And delighting in the uncertainty-rejoicing in it-spontaneous and full of surprises. You are a rich God. The certainty is your presence with us and in us. You don't "control" the world. And the world knows us not. But you are victorious over the world. And we can be certain that you will stay with us and transform us into a likeness of you.

15
Living Life to the Fullest

I think the truly amazing thing about Pete Nadherny during his illness was one simple thing: Pete never made his brain tumor, and the chance of its recurrence, the center of his life. He wasn't interested in researching information about his medical condition; he was much more interested in going fishing. He didn't read anything about brain tumors; he read about cars and boats and wine. His brain tumor became the center of my attention, but not his. As his physical health returned, his attention moved to all the things he wanted to do, and all the things he wanted to enjoy. As the organized business person he was, Pete started a list. His monthly MRI was just an interruption to him. We scheduled our travels around it.

Pete wrote his list on yellow legal paper. He dated the list with the month and year, and then he filed it in the magazine rack next to his favorite chair. The magazine rack had become his desk. He had things on that list that needed doing on the boat, the cars, and the house. He had things he wanted to buy on that list and places he wanted to go. His monthly meetings made his list. He loved checking things off.

The first thing on his list was to see both sons. We made the trip to Washington, DC to see Steve and Kathy first. The trip gave Pete a big happiness boost. Steve took us fishing on the Potomac River in a small rowboat with an electric motor. Pete's balance was challenged in getting in and out of the boat. He managed to throw out his own fishing line. He did great. But he also didn't move from his seat once

147

he got settled in the boat. He was like a fixture. He and Steve were both sad when we didn't catch any fish that day.

Pete managed to navigate the steep steps up to Steve and Kathy's guest bedroom and down to the basement several times while we were visiting. I was worried about his ankles swelling during the long trip in the car. We would stop at two- to three-hour intervals at a rest stop to walk around a little, which became a habit during our future travels. His left hand was still swollen a little, and he was still on Fla-gyl for that awful diarrhea, but we were on the final two weeks as the doctor tapered him off. Wine was soon to become a regular treat.

Shortly after the trip to D.C. to see Steve and Kathy, we headed to Florida to see Michael. Pete loved to have things to look forward to. Dinners out. Ballgames. The boat. And travel. One afternoon, Pete and I had lunch with two of my banker friends.

They blessed us by telling Pete, "You are such an inspiration to us and so many others. Perhaps that is your purpose."

Jenny said to Pete, "You remind us that love and family are the most important things. It helps me keep my job at the bank in per-spective, and urges me to do the things that are important—like your desire to visit Mount Rushmore!"

Pete laughed so hard during that lunch. Jenny and Greg were cre-ative and fun people. We talked politics and business and TV shows. Pete loved the energy during these lunches. He told them as we left, "We owe you the next one!"

Right before we left to see Michael in Florida, Pete piloted his boat for the first time since he had been diagnosed. Craig came with us, just in case. Pete handled the boat perfectly. Got in and out of the slip smoothly. He piloted the boat downtown, passing in front of our house on the river. He had been looking down on that river for so many days and nights, it was now fun for him to look up and see our house. He was on the river, captaining our boat without assistance! I was so proud of him, and so happy for him.

Pete was not afraid. He felt like he could do anything or go any-where. Although a cautious man, he was not going to let his brain tumor and its effects make him live in fear. He would push and stretch himself as far as he could. And I was his buddy, and being a risk-taker myself, our adventures had begun! He could drive our cars and pilot his boat. For Pete, it didn't get any better than this!

We went on our first real vacation on June 26, 2006. We drove the new station wagon on our own endurance race, traveling one thou-sand, nine hundred and forty-one miles to Florida and back. We made an initial stop in Atlanta, Georgia, and had dinner with our boat friend Craig, who worked in Atlanta. Pete drove through the busy Buckhead neighborhood, and managed to find the hotel just fine. All told, Pete drove about a third of this trip.

From Atlanta, we drove to St. Augustine. We hit Jacksonville on I-95 just as rush hour began. I asked him if he wanted to switch. He shook his head "No" and kept on. There were several instances that called for fast response times. I felt myself squirming a little, but didn't say a word. I could feel Pete's tension and concentration, but he didn't say a word. He didn't flinch. He sailed us through!

St. Augustine was a delight. It was my first visit. We stayed in an old historic hotel, the Casa Monica, which was in the heart of the old historic downtown. We walked to shops and dining, though we went slowly, and didn't go too far at any one outing. The Casa Monica had beach privileges at the Serenta Beach Club, so Pete and I did what we had done for years on vacations, spend afternoons on the beach and at the pool. Pete went swimming for the first time in the pool, while I headed to the ocean.

Michael had arranged for us to meet him and his girlfriend at Daytona for Brumo's Porsche 250-mile sports car race on June 29. Since we had missed the Daytona twenty-four-hour endurance sports car race at the end of January that year, getting to Daytona for a sports car race was particularly sweet for Pete. Michael knew how much it would mean to his father, which was why he had arranged everything. The presence of his son, and meeting his girlfriend who we liked a lot, made the race extra nice. Pete had always hoped Michael would meet someone else that he could love since his first marriage had ended years ago. We had met lots of girlfriends over the years, but this Jen was special to Michael, and Pete's hope for Michael's future happiness was kindled anew.

On the way home, we wound our way to our good friends, Jack and Judith, in McCormick, South Carolina. We spent the night catching up with each other. They had rented a pontoon boat for a trip out on Savannah Lake the next day. Pete laid himself out in the boat in the sun, enjoying the ride. Jack knew how much Pete loved being on the water. So many people loving us and supporting our journey. We took sustenance from them.

We then drove the nine-hour trip back to Cincinnati, and made it safely home by July 4. On the night of the Fourth, we sat on our deck and watched the hundreds of neighborhood fireworks displays in the hills across the river showing the "Best of America" tradition in this Midwestern town. It was glorious. And we were full of thanks.

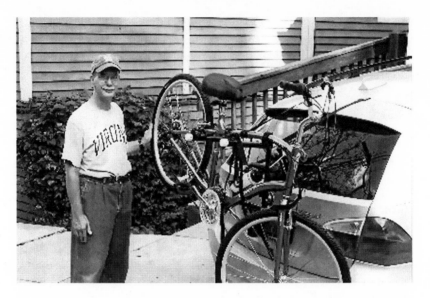

Pete and his bike

Pete's Carepage: August 3, 2006 @ 4:52 p.m.

I haven't updated for a while. This means things are very good for Pete and me. If we experience any change or difficulty, you will be the first to know. We count on your heightened level of prayer.

After seeing his two sons, Mike and Steve, Pete's next desire was to get to Chicago to see his family. We made the trip by "station wagon," and if you haven't driven to Chicago in a while the construction is "horrendouser" than usual as we tried to make our way to the Tri-State—Yikes! It looks like a war zone where 1–294, I-90 and I-80 converge. Everything is torn up and only two lanes going north or south just doesn't let traffic move very fast. Beware!

But other than the traffic it was a great visit. Pete drove a good part of the way. We saw his Aunt Vi and all the cousins. We must have had twenty people at dinner, many we had not seen in many years. So thank you, Chicago family, for all the love! Pete also got to visit his college roommate Larry and wife Cheryl in Joliet on the way home. Cheryl is also a medical miracle and Larry her caregiver, so we felt pretty privileged to be with these two miracle people—Pete and Cheryl!

Pete continues to get stronger. He is now walking a mile a day. His language and word recognition have taken a good "leap" and our speech therapist, Jenny, and I notice that Pete is using more complex sentence structure, and his reading comprehension is better. His handwriting looks like it used to look before he got sick! His hair is starting to grow out, the scars are healing and just yesterday, after a visit to his barber, he stopped wearing his hat 100 percent of the time. He left his hat off with Mike and Nan and Bill. A BIG deal! Bill continues to do healing touch on Pete weekly, and he and Nan's faithfulness is too much for words! Bill says Pete's energy fields are very "high," which means Pete's body is busy healing itself very nicely. One last accomplishment—last Saturday, Pete rode a bike! We went to the local bike trail and he got on his new bike and just rode and rode! Got pretty tired after a mile, but his balance didn't fail him. I was a little apprehensive—oh me of little faith!

Next big trip we are planning is to see my brother Joe and his wife Nancy. Joe promised Pete a salmon fishing trip if Pete recovered enough to do it. Pete has always wanted to catch a salmon. Sooo— September means salmon fishing!

P.S. Pete's next MRI will be August 6. I'll update again then. We count on all of your continued prayers for Pete's recovery. We trust that God will continue the glorious work he has begun in him. And I do believe it is the power of all of you asking and giving thanks that makes the difference. Thank YOU.

Family visits were now behind us. "What's next?" Pete asked me. We had initially talked about getting to Oregon for that salmon fishing trip with my brother by flying into South Dakota to see Mount Rushmore, and then driving through Wyoming to visit Yellowstone en route to Oregon. We got the map out, and used a highlighter to look at our plan.

Pete balked. His enthusiasm for the trip dwindled. "Three weeks is a long trip," he said. "Lots of driving. Too much."

I didn't argue. We bagged it.

But as the dog days of August settled into Cincinnati, we decided we could still visit all those places—but just do one place at a time. So on the spur of the moment, we decided to do part of our dream trip that week. We had a free week, which meant no doctor appointments and no tests required, so off we went to South Dakota.

Pete had been begging me for years to plan a trip to Mount Rushmore. He had always wanted to see it. I had been less than enthusiastic. In fact, I remember telling him that I had already seen Mount Rushmore. I was on the corporate jet with my boss on a trip from the

Twin Cities to Los Angeles. It was a clear day and Richard, knowing Pete's desire to see Mount Rushmore, pointed it out to me as we flew over. It was a beautiful white speck from fifteen thousand feet. I teased Pete when I returned that I had already been. You only needed to see Mount Rushmore once!

But off we went. We flew into Rapid City, South Dakota, and on the advice of Nan and Bill stayed in Custer State Park, where we could make the trip to Rushmore in less than an hour. The park was fantastic! We stayed in the lodge where Calvin Coolidge used to stay, ate buffalo for dinner and other wild game dishes we couldn't find in Ohio. We tried a different lodge dining room each night.

There were over fifteen hundred buffalo in the park and, in fact, as we tried to get to the lodge to check in, we had to stop the car to let the buffalo cross the road to their favorite watering hole. Pete was ecstatic. He loved animals of all kinds, and to see them in the wild and up close was a thrill. We met buffalo as we walked to the visitor center. We tracked them in the car on the loop around the park. We took their picture. We did a drive through a wildlife park with hundreds of bear, grey wolves and white wolves, reindeer, miniature ponies and mountain sheep. The bear came right up to the car. We hastily closed the windows.

Pete had bought a book years ago called the *Most Scenic Drives in America.* Two of those drives were right where we were staying. We traveled Needles Highway, which had cathedral-like rock formations in the Black Hills National Forest. We found a favorite road called Iron Mountain Road. It was a curvy, fifteen-miles-per-hour mountain pass on the way to Rushmore that had single-lane bridges and lots of wildlife. I would drive. Pete would scout for animals: wild turkeys and elk. White-tailed deer. I had not remembered seeing him so happy. He was like a kid with a new toy. And, oh yes, we did see Mount Rushmore. And the Crazy Horse memorial. We went for the day and stayed for the night lighting ceremony at Rushmore, which stirred patriotic feelings in both of us. But Pete was done. He had seen it. The wildlife scouting was a lot more fun for him than visiting the monument.

Pete remembered my birthday that September. I couldn't believe he remembered it. Steve and Kathy had sent us a couple dozen blue crabs from Maryland for our birthdays, so Pete and I covered our kitchen table in brown paper. We picked crabs and drank beer for hours to celebrate. Pete also made zucchini bread, one of his favorite things. He remembered how. And he remembered to take out the dry cleaning on

Tuesday nights. He wrote three short letters to friends! All new behaviors since he was sick; all normal things he did before he was sick.

Pete weighed in at 153 pounds. up from his low of 139 pounds. His weight before surgery was 169 pounds. Pete stopped taking naps, and right before we left to go to Oregon, Pete climbed into our red Porsche convertible and took it for a spin. The Porsche had a clutch. It was the first time he had taken this car out since surgery. I was with him and let out a loud "whoo-hoo!" into the air.

The flight from Cincinnati to Portland, Oregon, is four hours and twenty minutes. Pete tolerated the air travel well, walking on his own and toting his roller-bag behind him through the airports. The first night we stayed at a hotel right on the Columbia River, and walked the flood wall watching all the boats and the gulls on a beautiful sunny afternoon with no humidity, and the river a wonderful blue. The next day Pete and I went exploring the Columbia River gulch and stopped at Multnomah Falls, marveling at the waterfall and having a salmon lunch at the lodge. Salmon always tastes better in the Northwest. We had dinner that first night with some US Banker friends at a restaurant on the river. Pete didn't know these people very well, but he showed no hesitation in visiting them. I don't know if he was doing it for me or whether he really enjoyed them. He was his usual gracious self, and had asked their names a couple of times as we drove to the restaurant.

The next morning we were off toward Bend, Oregon, taking Route 26 east from the city, following it up the hill to Government Camp and Timber Lodge at Mount Hood, then down through the canyon of the Warm Springs Indian Reservation and south to Bend. We had visited Abby and Dick the year before Pete's diagnosis, and had taken a long hike up to Broken Top Mountain where Pete walked in the snow. This year would be different. No long hikes. Rather, it was a drive in the car to the Cascades and the Deschutes National Forest riding by Batchelder Mountain.

Pete loved Dick. Former neighbors, Dick was a man's man, having served as a secret service agent for a number of presidents. He was a conservative Republican, and Pete and Dick loved talking politics and history. Dick's new vocation was a rescuer for people getting lost or injured in the mountains around Bend. He was studying hard while we were there, and Pete loved asking him questions about what he was learning about physiology and safety.

While Pete took a nap at their home, Abby, Dick and I got into a long conversation about spirituality and faith. Abby is Jewish, and had been serious about her own spiritual journey for a long time. I shared what I was learning around my own journey since being Pete's caregiver. Abby asked me what Pete's faith was like. I had just asked Pete that question while on the plane flying out. I shared with them what Pete told me. "I believe in God and that belief has gotten a lot more and deeper recently. I want to help others," he kept repeating. "Do anything I can to help others. And to keep a positive attitude. Whatever will be, I accept."

Pete never said once, the whole time I cared for him, that he was sick. I would use the word—"since you got sick"—but Pete never used the term. Pete played a mean game of bocce ball that night in the park next to the Deschutes River, across the street from Dick and Abby's home. Pete won a few games. The look on his face of utter concentration will stay in my memory for a long time.

My brother Joe had lined up a guide to take us salmon fishing. We were right on the edge of the end of the salmon fishing season on the Columbia River. Pete and I both knew we risked missing the season altogether by going this late, but couldn't leave for the trip earlier in September because Mike was having thyroid surgery in Cincinnati. Pete wouldn't leave town until he knew Mike was okay. The plan was to meet Joe and Nancy, his wife, at their home in Eugene, and head out to fish from there.

We drove out of Bend over the summit of McKenzie Pass in the Willamette National Forest at over five thousand feet elevation. The temperature dropped, and the scenery changed to a harsh, black, shiny volcanic rock. It was snowing on the pass. So much for the Mustang convertible we had rented! Pete stayed in the car with the heater running, as I stopped and ran to the top of the Dee Wright Observatory. Such an odd, old, harsh beauty at that pass.

By the time we got to Eugene, the guide had called Joe and said that the Oregon Fish and Wildlife Department had just closed the Columbia River for salmon fishing. So plans changed. Instead of heading to Portland, we were heading to the Oregon coast to fish for salmon on the Aquinas River in Newport. We got up before dawn for the two-hour drive to the coast from Eugene. We saw the sunrise on the Aquinas at 6:45 a.m. It was a sparkling silver and grey sun behind the mist that hung low on the river. Pete had laid out six layers of clothes on the floor the night before. Once at the marina he put on all six shirts, along with the knit cap that Nancy had knitted for him, complete with a silver salmon fish pin. Nancy had sent that knit cap to Pete while he was recovering from the surgery at Cleveland Clinic in

January. Each loop had been knit in love, with the hope that one day Pete could wear it while he fished for salmon. And here he was, posing with Nancy's hat on for a picture.

Pete's Carepage: September 16, 2006 @ 3:32 p.m.

We are updating our Carepage from warm and balmy Oregon! We could tell you a fish story about how we caught 121 Dungeness crab and 121 salmon but we only took a picture of the crab and not the salmon, but we know you wouldn't believe it. So the truth is we fished all morning for salmon and couldn't get a bite (neither could the other fishermen), so we turned to crabbing in the afternoon and we did catch 121 Dungeness and had "26 keepers" which we then brought home, cleaned and had a crab feast for dinner and crab and eggs for breakfast! The good news is it didn't rain as forecasted but it

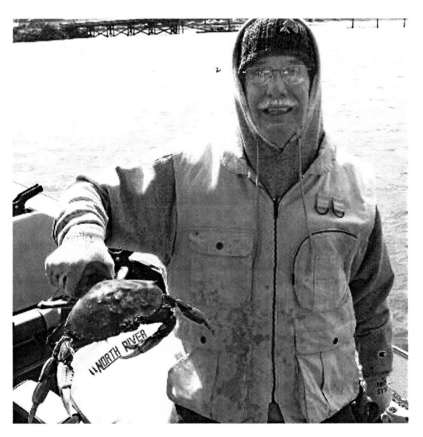

Pete in his salmon fishing hat, with a crab catch

was cold (Pete had on six layers of shirts and jackets) AND the sun
was out, so we had a lot of fun. Pete ate all the brownies while on the
boat and says "guess we have to come back next year and get that
salmon!"

Pete turned sixty-one in late September, after we got back home. I
gave Pete his birthday gifts at breakfast. I got him a fishing pole and
net. He was so excited. He played with that pole in our living room,
acting like he was casting. We both cried when he opened his card
that played "Let's Spend the Night Together," one of his all-time
favorite songs. We biked and shopped and had a nice dinner out. A
playful day. Just perfect.

Pete began to use his fishing pole. He and I headed out to a local
lake where we could buy bait and Pete could get down to the water
safely. When Pete and I went fishing we never caught anything. That
was okay for me because I just enjoyed being out in the sun and near
the water, but I don't think it was okay for Pete. He'd get frustrated.
He'd try different bait and different spots. Thank goodness for our
Crossroads small-group friend, Matt.

Pete complained in our small group about not being able to catch
any fish. Matt who is an expert fisherman, took Pete out fishing with
him one October morning. Pete had to get up early, meeting Matt near
the Ohio River by 6:45. Matt had an old fishing boat with an outboard
motor. He'd take it where the little Miami and the Ohio rivers converge, and drop bait on lines fishing off the bottom. I'll never forget
Pete coming home that morning. He smelled like the river itself, and
he was clammy and muddy.

"I caught the biggest fish Matt has ever caught on the Ohio! It was
thirty-five pounds," Pete said, extending his arms to show how big it
was. "Matt had a scale on his boat, and he weighed the fish before we
threw it back in. Matt had a few lines in the water and Matt caught a
fish; then it was my turn and I caught a fish. Matt caught another one
and then my line dipped way down, and Matt and I both knew we had
a big one," Pete told me excitedly. Pete looked like he was six years
old. His eyes were glistening, and he was smiling the biggest smile I
had seen in a long time.

By now, we had made a significant dent in Pete's list. We had been
to Washington DC and Florida to see both sons. We made it back to
Daytona for a sports car race. We had visited Pete's family in Chicago. We had seen Mount Rushmore. We had been fishing a number
of times and he even had caught a big one. And we had made it to

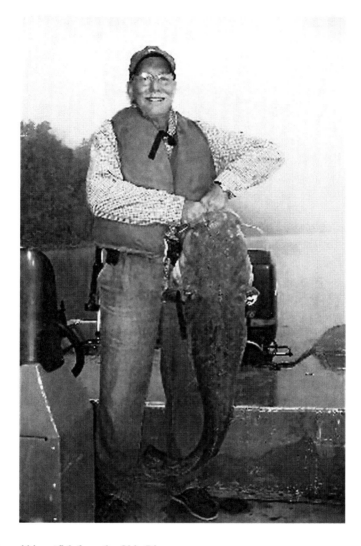

Pete and his catfish from the Ohio River

Oregon to go salmon fishing. We were approaching Pete's one-year anniversary from diagnosis. WOW!

As winter approached, Pete kept getting better. He went into his office at the Angus Group for the monthly sales meetings. He initiated calls to the electrician, the deck cleaning service, the fish market and more. He started remembering things that he had committed to previously with other people, and was following through without prompting. He made a new to-do list and started working it. He was remembering all the routines of the week: the day for garbage, dry cleaning, house cleaners. He took the car out for gas and picked up pictures on his own while I was at a meeting. He calendared and attended all his board meetings: the two charter schools; Hillside Trust; Mount Adams Civic Association and his Chamber CEO Roundtable meetings. He seemed to really enjoy the meetings and was engaged from what he would report back to me. One day, he got the ladder out and cleaned the gutters. Talk about having his balance back! His humor and sarcasm were back, too.

The Rolling Stones were coming to Louisville, Kentucky at the end of September. Pete had spied the notice in early August in the Cincinnati paper, and called immediately for tickets. This was right in the middle of one of those scares when we were uncertain if the tumor had returned or not. Pete didn't show any caution. Whether he would be well enough to go to the Stones concert wasn't even a consideration. "Let's call and get tickets now," he said. And he did.

That was Pete's reaction to his illness. He couldn't really ignore it; there were too many doctor visits and pills to take, but his illness didn't control his decisions about what he wanted to do and how he wanted to live. He didn't let the threat of brain cancer control his life. Pete loved the Stones. They were his favorite musical group. He had every CD from every US concert. He had the collection *Stones Singles: The London Years.* He had the "Four Flicks," DVDs of some of the Stones' live concerts. He had a Rolling Stones T-shirt with the big, red tongue plastered on his chest. We had seen them perform live in Cincinnati and in Washington, DC. Now the Rolling Stones were performing an historic first at Churchill Downs.

We went down by ourselves and checked into the hotel after a late lunch in our favorite neighborhood in Louisville. During the concert, the rain came down. It poured. It didn't matter. There was Pete in the stands with thousands of his closest friends, drenched and cheering wildly at all his favorite songs only seven months after brain surgery.

Since Pete and I had quit working, we had a good opportunity to volunteer together somewhere. Pete had his community commitments: the two charter school boards, the Hillside Trust, the CEO Roundtable and the chamber. I had my commitments: the YWCA and the United Way. We volunteered together at Crossroads, but that was it. So we developed a list of organizations where we might find a volunteer role together, doing something we both had a passion for.

We met first with the executive director of the City Gospel Mission, a shelter for the homeless in a very poor neighborhood, Over-the-Rhine, in Cincinnati. Pete had done some work with this executive director in the past. There was opportunity at City Gospel, but the executive director was encouraging us to volunteer in order to build long-term relationships with his clients, and not just do a project. We didn't rule this opportunity out, but wanted to pursue some other options first.

Our next appointment was with the CEO of the YWCA, Charlene Ventura. Pete had worked with Charlene on some search assignments, and actually placed her program director. I had been honored by the YWCA as a Career Woman of Achievement, and had joined the YWCA Board in 2004. Charlene jumped at the chance to utilize Pete and me.

In a short time Pete and I were designing a training program for leadership development for the YWCA "Rising Stars," prospective young women leaders in the community. Pete and I both had human resource and training backgrounds, so we felt comfortable with the assignment. Funding got approved for the project in the fall from a local foundation. Many a day we would go to therapy in the mornings, and be at the YWCA in the afternoons. I was impressed by Pete's stamina. He was generally quiet at the meetings, but he had his portfolio out and would occasionally take notes. He'd make suggestions as to what we should include in the program design. After a series of meetings that we conducted at the YWCA, and lots of discussion at home between the two of us, we designed the program, launching it in January of 2007 for about forty of the "Rising Stars" in Cincinnati.

"Tall Stacks" came to Cincinnati in early October of 2006. Tall Stacks was a week-long festival of riverboats that gathered together from all over the Midwest every four years or so. Cincinnati was founded as a riverboat town, so it was always a grand celebration when the boats arrived. Our home looked out on the Ohio River. For a week we had a regular parade of riverboats.

We enjoyed this year of Tall Stacks more than any previous years, because we weren't working. We walked down and attended the festival three days in a row, even going out one day on our boat to get a close-up view. It was a beautiful weather week, with 75-degree days and clear nights. Pete and I sat on the river wall, listened to a concert and enjoyed watching all the boats and activity. That night when we got home we sat on our deck with a glass of wine and Pete lit his first cigar since surgery last January. Ahh, contentment!

We had talked about having a party during Tall Stacks for those who had been so kind to us through the last months. Our house, overlooking the Ohio River, was a perfect place to view the boats. Pete loved hosting parties. He loved the planning, and he was an active partner in both the preparation and the execution. He ordered enough prime rib to feed an army. He cooked it carefully to perfection, and carved it with tenderness. We had fresh shrimp and smoked salmon. Lots of wine. It was a feast for all of our neighbors and friends.

The party was on Sunday afternoon, timed to allow our guests a view of the major event of the week, the Tall Stacks Grand Parade. We watched *The Colonel* from Galveston, Texas; the *Spirit of Peoria,* an authentic paddle wheeler; *The Natchez* from New Orleans; the *Harriett Bishop* from St. Paul. The *Jackson* from Nashville led the way for the two grand dames, the *Delta* and *Mississippi Queens.* It was a glorious day. The calliope was playing, and the music was drifting up to our deck. By nightfall, there was a harvest moon rising. Pete was the consummate host, welcoming each person to our home, and making sure everything was just right on the table. I loved Pete as much that day as any. He was so delighted to entertain those he loved and cared about.

When we were planning the party, Pete and I had an argument over who to invite. Family or friends or both? Pete wanted only friends invited, plus Mary Jo and Mike; I wanted friends and family. He was adamant against it. Pete wanted what he wanted. I wanted what I wanted. I pulled the trump card, like I had done so many times in our past, when I didn't get my way. "We just won't do the party at all since we can't agree," I stubbornly pronounced. Such tension between us. Pete waited patiently.

I quickly recognized how ugly my anger and resentment was. I had recently been influenced by Greg Boyd, a theologian and author introduced to us at Crossroads. He provided a definition of love that made so much sense to me that it became my touchstone for all that I did. "Love is ascribing unsurpassable worth to others at cost to ourselves." It was not love if it didn't cost something. I realized how wrong I was to throw a tantrum over one event. Such a small thing. How could I believe in this definition of love, and not give up what I wanted? And to give it up in a way that there was true joy between Pete and I, and not a festering resentment and tension as we prepared for the party. I gave up what I wanted; that is, not the party. And what I had been so stubborn about really did disappear. I didn't think about it again. Funny how big concepts, like love, get tested in the small, routine things. The party was a joyful occasion.

I worried a little that Pete and I were having too much fun. Pete and I talked about what we should be doing for others. I want to "start working more in religion," Pete would say. I wasn't sure what that meant to him, but would listen for ways to translate that desire of his. I asked him at one point if he wanted to join the mentoring project at Crossroads to help job hunters get work. I thought that would be something he would be well suited for, and would jump at the chance. I would have joined him. But he said "No." Guess that was not what he had in mind. I followed his lead.

Near the top of Pete's list was getting the bathrooms fixed. We had three bathrooms in our home. The original tile installer had done a bad job, and for years tiles had popped up and cracked periodically. Pete would repair them, but it drove him crazy. He had a real urgency about getting these bathrooms re-done now. He asked one of his Roundtable members, who owned and ran a construction company, if he was interested in the job. Drew said yes.

Pete was excited. We engaged an architect because we were moving some walls in the master bathroom to expand the closet and dressing area. We had the hot tub removed, which we had used once in thirteen years, and tripled the size of our shower. After showering for all those years in a small dark shower where both my elbows touched the walls when I washed my hair, I had fantasies of wild orgies in this new shower. Pete and I could easily get in this shower together— along with a shower chair. Oh, well, the fantasies of the orgies were just that.

We met with the architect in October. We shopped and shopped, picking out the right marble for the floor and walls, the right granite for the sinks. Then the fixtures and the tile and the paint. We shopped as if on an all-important mission, making decisions quickly and with little angst. By the beginning of November, the work was started. It was all done by Christmas. For sixty days, we lived in construction dust with workmen as family members. Our clothes were hung on temporary hanging racks that Pete had rented. It was chaos as home construction always was. Only been nine months before, Pete had been in intensive care and nearly died. Now he was the construction manager! And he didn't seem bothered at all by all the disruption.

Pete wanted to get our house remodeled for me! That's what was causing his sense of urgency. He didn't know how much time he had left. "I want it just fine for you," Pete said. "So when I am gone, it will be perfect for you!"

Tears filled my eyes. I was so loved. He was doing all this for me! "Will you sell the house?" Pete asked.

"No way!" I said.

"Well, if you do at some point, then maybe you will get more value out of it."

I was dumbstruck. The silence sat between us like a tender friend.

One day at breakfast during the construction, Pete told me he thought about his death every day when he woke up. He told me that he searched for words to pray, but could not always find them. I thought about how fond the Lord must be of Pete. How He must look into his heart, and see so much love, even when Pete's words failed him. One day Pete asked me to look up and print some prayers for him. I got on the internet and asked him to join me. He asked me to print the Lord's Prayer, the Apostle's Creed and the Hail Mary. Pete carefully cut out those prayers and taped them all on a piece of cardboard, which he carefully covered with one of the plastic sleeves he always used for important documents. He put those prayers in his newly converted magazine rack/desk next to his chair.

We didn't let the construction get in the way of having more fun. We went to Keeneland Race Track in Lexington, Kentucky one fall day with Mary Jo and Mike, and included in the trip a visit to one of Kentucky's bourbon distilleries, Woodford Reserve, an old historic distillery nestled in the hills of Kentucky. We enjoyed the smells of the casks, the historic buildings, the grounds and the bourbon tasting. We drove the back roads over to the track and saw some of the most beautiful horse farms in the world.

Mike started sharing some of his memories of his father, who loved horses so much. Mike loved horses because of his dad, and could feel his dad's presence with him, especially at the track. Pete shared more about the loss of his parents then he had ever shared before with anyone other than me. He talked about his dad dying while he was at school.

"How naïve I was," Pete said. "I had no idea that my dad was that sick. He died at home. I didn't even get to tell him good-bye."

Then, three short years later, Pete was doing his homework at home, and his mother collapsed in the bathroom from an apparent heart attack. Pete ran to her. She wouldn't move. Pete called 911. She was gone. Pete, a young boy, left all alone. No siblings. What feelings of abandonment he must have had. He grew up fast.

At Keeneland, Pete was intent on winning. He read and studied the racing program, doing his calculations on which horse to bet on for each race. He was so intent. He was reading and understanding! I loved watching his face, and his logical mind making all those connections: past winning history, jockey's record and the odds.

Before each race began, we walked right up to the guardrail of the track. You could smell the mud from there and see it fly from the horses' hooves. Pete would scream, "Go four!" or "Go one!" or "Go three! Come on! Go! Go! You can do it!" His excitement was so high. When his horse won, he'd go in and cash his ticket, kind of secretive about how much money he had won. And Pete was a winner that day! He picked a winner in every race of the day. He came home with money in his pocket and had had a good time. That was Pete's criteria for a good day at the races.

Pete's Carepage: December 8, 2006 @ 4:35 p.m.

More GOOD NEWS! Pete had his latest MRI and doc visit yesterday, and there is still no sign of any kind of tumor activity or cancer present. WHOO-HOO! The injured area is still there but it was a little smaller than it was thirty days ago, improved enough that the doc cut Pete's steroid dosage in half. Praise God again. His power is so evident. And thanks to all of you for your continued prayer, belief in Pete, unrelenting requests for his healing and your support of me. What a GREAT Christmas present we have received. Another "no worry zone" straight through the holidays!

Since our last update, Pete and I have been in a "Thanksgiving mode." He told me the other day, "I give thanks each morning when I wake up—just for breathing!" From Pete's and my perspective there are no bad days. And we have had lots of good ones! We made it to Florida again getting great visits with son Mike and family, Jen and Chelsea. We got a boat ride in the wonderful waters around Clearwater with Pete's best friend Jerry, and re-connected with old friends, the Silvestris, who we hadn't seen in over ten years. They just moved to St. Petersburg from Philadelphia. The weather cooperated, giving us 82 degrees and sunny every day, which sounds pretty good today, with temps in Ohio hovering around 20 degrees. We drove to Clearwater with Pete driving seventy-five percent of the way. We needed an excuse to break the trip up on the way home, and my sister Mary Jo and Mike happened to be in Hilton Head on business that weekend, so we had to stop. Had a wonderful weekend. Pete rode his bike on the beach, which exhausted him. He decided bike trails were friendlier. He even spied an alligator sunning himself along the side of the trail. Went fishing in the backwater of Hilton head and Pete was jealous when Mike brought in a twenty-six-inch redfish and he ended the day empty-handed. Nothing like the sunsets in Hilton Head!

So Pete and I are doing better than fine! We are doing our first volunteer community project together, designing a board leadership training program with a special emphasis on racial justice/gender equity for the greater Cincinnati YWCA "up and coming" women. Great fun for Pete and me to be in meetings together. Pete does well. Makes his contribution and stays with the conversation which is fast and long. Last night, I asked him to join me at the zoo with the United Way staff and nineteen kids and single moms at the Christmas Festival of Lights. It was about fourteen degrees and Pete was the only guy. He was a life-saver for all the five-year-old boys who needed to find a bathroom!

This Christmas will be a special one for both of us. Both sons and their families will be coming to Cincinnati to celebrate with us. We will be spending New Year's Eve this year in Phoenix with our friends from Boston and South Carolina, marking the fifteenth consecutive year of an NYE tradition.

Today as I write this it is almost exactly one year from the date of Pete's diagnosis. As Pete says, with great glee, "They gave me only six months and look at me now!" Okay, Pete, we are looking at you now, buddy! Admiring your courage and humbly thanking God for the miracles he has performed in you! We give thanks to all of you who have followed us on this journey for the last twelve months. YOU are amazing in your faithfulness and love. We couldn't have asked God for a better set of "arms and legs" than the ones you have given us. Thanks. Have a wonderful holiday!

The year was ending and the Christmas holidays were upon us. Christmas was always special, even more so when the kids, Michael and Steve and Kathy would come in. They didn't make visits home a routine for Christmas, although we had shared many of them together. Pete and I surely didn't pressure them, but when they were here, it was extra nice!

This year, shortly after Thanksgiving, Pete told me, "I'm not sure for how many more Christmases I'll be here. I'd love the guys to be home, even if I have to pay to get them here."

I felt my heart break within me. It brought up lots of old memories of times when they had ignored their father's desires.

"You should probably make sure they know that you really want them to come home this year. Maybe send a note or call them," I said.

"I gave them a hint when we called them Thanksgiving Day," he said.

"Do you want me to send them a note letting them know how much that would mean to you?" I asked him.

"No, not yet." Pete said. "I'll think about it."

In my prayer journal I asked God to send an angel message ever-so-lightly to the guys. How I wanted his desire satisfied! I thought about acting on my own—that would be typical of me, just to do it. But I didn't. I honored Pete's request.

We made an overnight trip to Nashville, Indiana, which was an artists' community set in the foothills of Brown County State Park. Pete and I had made this trip many, many years before as our way of getting in the Christmas mood. Tiny white pin lights adorned the main street of the village, perched on a steep hill, Christmas decorations, many hand-crafted and unique, were everywhere. We shopped all our favorite places and enjoyed the best fried chicken in the world at the General Store. I was so thankful that another trip to Nashville was possible.

When we got home, Steven called. Pete always wanted me to be right next to him when the guys called. It gave him more confidence in case he had a word-finding challenge. I was looking at his face, and saw tears of joy welling up in his eyes. "They are coming home," Pete said after hanging up. "And I didn't have to call them. They are coming home on their own."

Michael brought Jen and her daughter Chelsea home with him for Christmas. Pete was delighted, and loved Chelsea instantly. Both Jen and Chelsea were beautiful women, and wonderfully warm and kind. Pete was into cameras for gifts this year. He bought Michael and Steve his very favorite red Casio camera that fit into a shirt pocket. Pete brought such intensity to these purchases. He was on a mission! We had to make an extra trip to find just the right model. No other brand or color would do. Once Pete gave them the cameras, it was Chelsea who could not put that camera down. She loved it and Pete was so delighted that someone else shared his passion for his Casio!

Pete went to his Angus group Christmas dinner party, and made the rounds like he was still the CEO. They were so glad to see him. He was so missed at the company. His legacy was deep with the business people in this city, his customers. One of his colleagues was gratefully telling me how great a year she'd had, as she picked up all the business from Pete's customers. "They all love him and ask about him," she said. Pete spoke at the dinner. I was surprised that he so readily spoke in public. He thanked them for the year. It was Pete's night.

A couple of days after Christmas, Pete started growing a goatee. He said he had always wanted to do it. I guess this was another thing on his list. Checked it: done. He was so delighted with himself. I loved the goatee. I smiled and smiled and kissed him on his new growth. A New Year was beginning, and Pete had a new look!

My prayer journal: New Year's Eve, 2006

2006 was a life-changing year. Life-changing means that nothing will ever be the same again. There is no going back. And so it is. I have learned so much more about you. Your presence has been with us. Your presence is enough.

We deepened the friendship with Nan and Bill. Pete benefited from Bill's Healing Touch. Mary Jo and Mike came crashing into our life with their commitment to walk with us. They are a daily presence.

You changed me. You rescued me from work; you convicted me of pride and judgment. I felt real fear this year. I felt totally out of control: Pete barely walking; Pete losing his speech; Pete sleeping for long periods of time and me dealing with the loneliness.

You have rescued Pete. You have fought for us. You have fought this awful disease in Pete. You sent your archangels! You have heard our cry for help and you have been full of mercy and grace. You have blessed this year with yourself. You have redeemed this year for us. And I thank you for your protection, your mercy, your grace.

I ask you to bless this coming year—2007. It is a year of new beginnings. For the first time in thirty years, I begin a year without work responsibilities and pressure. My mission is to care for Pete. It is a challenging mission. I want to honor you in doing it. Let us witness faithfully to you through our love of each other.

16

Pete: The Endurance Race Car Driver

Pete and I were blessed with good and faithful friends. We had a tradition of spending each New Year's with two other couples in a different city each year. In 2006, Pete and I had shared his diagnosis with these same friends in the bar of a hotel in Charleston, South Carolina. Now, after two brain surgeries, hospitalization to fight his bout with pneumonia, hospitalization to deal with blood clots, months of physical, occupational and speech therapies, fifteen MRIs, six weeks of radiation treatments, changes in both of our careers and work life, facing death and living with uncertainty, the six of us were together again marking the fifteenth year we celebrated New Year's together. This year, 2007 found us in Phoenix, Arizona. It was cold in Phoenix; the hotel covered the flowers with sheets at night to keep them from freezing. I was just thankful to make this trip. How comforting it was for me for the six of us to be together again.

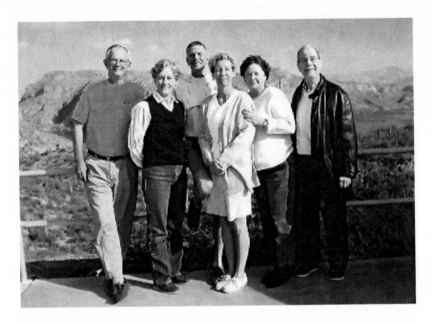

Pete and our New Year's friends in Phoenix

Pete's Carepage: January 11, 2007 @ 5:51 p.m.

Happy New Year! Here we are with our friends Mike and Pam from Boston and Jack and Judith from South Carolina, on the Apache Trail right outside of Phoenix. We had a great New Year—our friends played golf and Pete and I managed a bike ride in the desert on New Year's Day, then all of us were guests at an gourmet dinner made by our bank friends Judie and Carl Carl gets all the credit for the cooking!) in beautiful Fountain Hills! What a GREAT way to start 2007!

GOOD NEWS continues. We got the results from Pete's latest MRI today and saw no change from December. Only "injury"; no signs of cancer or tumor. In fact, for the first time Pete doesn't have to go back for another MRI for six weeks vs. the every-thirty-days schedule we have been on. Progress! It is now over a year since Pete's diagnosis, and Pete's greatest concern right now is whether his newly grown "goatee" (two weeks old) will fill out and look good! Oh my!

Christmas was the best ever! Mike and his girlfriend Jen and daughter Chelsea from the Tampa area, and Steve and Kathy from DC area were both in to celebrate. Pete was beaming! And then the Beechem clan descended on our house for the traditional Christmas Day night fare with Scattergories and puzzles and a hot game of euchre where Mom Beechem cleaned up!

We continue to give thanks and praise for God's healing in Pete. The Cleveland Clinic and our Cincinnati doctor are working closely together, which is so reassuring to us, and we add this cooperation to the "miracle" list. Bill and Nan are our ever-faithful "healers" and are still doing "healing touch" on Pete once a week. This is their one-year anniversary, too! How blessed we are to have them. Bill is working with Pete now, with essential oils that increase the power of the healing. In fact, last week Bill had the most powerful healing session yet. There was so much energy in our house—WOW! God continues to do awesome work as Pete moves to full recovery. So we are blessed and very happy. We thank all of you who continue to remember us and pray for Pete—your "lifting us up" in prayer faithfully has been the source of healing power. Our hope for each of you is a deep and rich and wonderful 2007.

The snow came a few days in January. Pete shoveled snow using a shovel and the snow blower for almost an hour. Then he took a long nap. We did normal things. Pete went to the Angus group for the monthly sales meeting. He attended his CEO Roundtable and charter school board meetings, and we worked hard on the YWCA Rising Star project, preparing for the first class to kick off in February. Bill visited once a week for his healing sessions with Pete. We met with our life group from Crossroads every Monday night. Pete made love to me many times that month. His only pleasure was in seeing me have pleasure. How loved I felt!

One day Pete was going to a Chamber of Commerce event at the University of Cincinnati Conference Center. He got lost on his way. I had asked him if he knew where he was going before he left. He said he did. I made a Google map for him, just in case. He called me from the car. I realized then how stupid I was. The words on the map naming streets were useless to Pete. He could not receive meaningful information in that form any longer. Pete finally made it to the Chamber event, but a trip that would normally take twenty minutes took him an hour and a half.

Big learning for me to change how Pete prepared to go out on his own. What worked for Pete, we learned, was to verbally review his course of driving together before he left the house, using landmarks that he knew, not street names. These landmarks would trigger in his memory the right course. "You'll pass the Shell station in Clifton, and then come to a 't' where the old Hughes High School was. Turn right. When you get to the corner where Dr. Smith's office is, turn right again," I'd say. Pete would nod in perfect understanding. The only time this approach didn't work was when I didn't know how to get to where he was going because I had not been there myself. Pete never seemed afraid of this situation. He'd go anyway. And one time, he never did find the destination after driving around for hours. He finally came home frustrated, but not deterred.

Pete was amazing at geography. He couldn't name the street, but his mind had lost none of its sharpness in knowing where he was going. In fact, when my sister was driving us somewhere, Pete would be telling her when to change lanes or where to turn to get to our destination. When he was driving by himself, my job was to give Pete a frame of reference so his mind, through pictures, not words, would remember where he was going, and once he remembered, he had no problem getting there. The very next day, after he got lost going to the Chamber meeting, he successfully traveled the fifty miles to and from our home for one of his CEO Roundtable meetings without any problem, because he could picture where he was going; he just couldn't name the streets to get there.

I learned some new things in January about myself. I was constantly changing and growing through my prayer time and interaction with Pete. Pete told me how much he resented me finishing his stories for him when we were with other people. Ouch! I was guilty as charged. Pete talked so slowly. His searching for words was painstaking, and I wondered if the listeners were tiring. My impatience would make me jump in and speed up the sharing. I did not give Pete the space and time to talk. How wrong of me. I asked Pete for forgiveness.

In examining that tendency, I saw my overall impatience had been fueled for years by my task habits. Do stuff. Do it fast. Do multiple tasks at one time. I suddenly saw how un-loving that behavior truly was. Being engaged with a person required listening. Really paying attention to Pete was the most loving thing I could do for both of us. I started taking more time after dinner just to sit at the table with Pete. I resisted the urge to get up and clean the table off, or start the dishes. I just sat. I had missed the chance so many times just to be with him. Pete noticed the change. He thanked me. He really appreciated this time, and it became a very special time for us right after our evening meal. He talked more than he had before. And I felt a deep joy. Our life group told Pete during that January that "he was a miracle in their midst." They were right.

On the fourth weekend in January every year, the Daytona International Speedway hosts the Rolex 24-Hour Sports Car Race. The race started at one p.m. on Saturday and finished at one p.m. on Sunday. The endurance of this race attracted Rolex to sponsor it for the last couple of years. There were usually about seventy cars that started, racing in four different classes, so in essence, you had four races happening simultaneously in the same race. Just to finish this race was bragging rights for the race year to come. Usually between thirty to forty cars finished.

The Daytona oval track that NASCAR used opened up into the infield for this race to a three-and-one-half-mile course, which weaved through eight infield turns and then back to the oval, where the drivers had the chance to purse very high speeds.

Pete had been going to this race since he lived in Jacksonville, Florida in the early Seventies. He rarely missed it. He had been to this race well over thirty times; I had been with him every year of our twenty-three-year marriage. Going to this race was one of the first things Pete and I did when we met. I had learned sports car racing from Pete, and learned to love this race. The twenty-four hours was a race with more Porsches competing, because it leveraged their endurance, speed and handling. This year we took Mary Jo and Mike to the race. Michael and Jen and family met us there.

It was a clear blue-sky day, at seventy degrees. For the one p.m. race start, Pete got us to the track by no later than eight-thirty a.m. to secure a good parking space in the infield. We made our breakfast trip to Krispy Kreme before we got to the track and Pete ordered his normal dozen doughnuts, which he subsequently ate with his first beer as soon as we parked. All part of the tradition, made especially sweet this year because he was here! We had listened to this race last year in the intensive care step-down unit at the Cleveland Clinic. While Pete was tethered to the pumps of the IL-13 trial, Steve and Mike had this race live on their laptops so Pete could listen. We were not sure then if we would ever get back. But here we were!

Pete loved showing Mike and Mary Jo around the track. It was their first time, and Pete was like a proud dad showing his kids his favorite place in the world. We visited the garage areas before the race began, walking right up to the cars, their drivers and mechanics. We walked out to the grid when all the cars lined up for the start, and snaked our way through the TV camera crews, fans like ourselves, and the driver teams. Pete walked them onto the oval so they could feel the steepness of the slope in the grade of the track. Mike exaggerated almost falling over from the slant. Pete laughed like a kid. The start of the race created such excitement! The roar of the engines and the smell of the oil. Nothing like it.

After the start, we walked. And we walked. From one vantage point in the infield to the next, we walked back and forth and back and forth, with the loud blaring of the engines in our ears and the dirt of the track in our teeth. Pete had supplied us all with ear radios for listening to the announcers amid the blare. The smell of the fuel was intoxicating for race car fans. Periodically, we'd walk back to the pits to watch the crews in action, as the cars would come in for fuel or tires or to change drivers, since each team had three to five drivers for the long twenty-four hours.

As the hours drew long, we'd sneak back to the garages and watch the crews fixing sick cars. In a twenty-four-hour race, a car could come back to the garage, get fixed, and still make it back to the track to compete. Pete was amazing at this race. Pete's stamina was so good, he wore us all out. By nightfall, we were ready for a dinner in a nice restaurant, a shower and bed in a nice hotel. The next morning we returned to the track to see the finish from the grandstand.

We made it home by early February. On Valentine's Day in 2007, Pete took me out to dinner. It was a week where his blood pressure had spiked dangerously high for no apparent reason, and we had spent all week taking his pressures and adjusting medicines. Pete never let his illness get in the way of the important things!

"It's Valentine's Day," he said. "We're going out." At dinner, Pete said, "I am changing so much. I want to live forever with God. I am getting closer to religion. I am amazed at Bill. The way he hears angels and God's speaking to him," Pete said, shaking his head. "I don't hear those things. Do you?" he asked.

I said "No way. Bill has a special gift."

"Well, I just want to help and do good for others," Pete said.

I was full of joy. I could see God doing His work in Pete. How blessed I was to witness this.

The next day Pete shared his frustration at my controlling attitude toward him. He got mad when I asked him if he had taken his pills. "You are always bugging me," he said, "like when you ask if I got ALL the garbage, even the stuff upstairs."

"You are right," I said. "I'll stop." That was the end of the conversation.

But I learned an important lesson. When Pete was feeling well, I needed to trust his judgment and decision-making, and stop second-guessing him. It was hard for me because sometimes Pete remembered, and sometimes he didn't. But usually I knew when I had to double-check stuff. I didn't need to give him that burden. He was a very independent man. I had to learn to respect that. How lucky I was to have this problem, I thought. Many in his situation would just have abdicated all responsibility for anything. Here was Pete, fighting me to trust him. After this conversation, we went and finished the taxes to prepare them for our accountant. Pete did the recording of expenses and calculated totals. He had a system he had used for many years for preparing our tax worksheet. I followed his lead. We enjoyed working together. Such joy. Taxes!

Sebring, Florida is about two and a half hours due south of Orlando. It has a race track and hosts the second endurance race in the country, "The 12 Hours of Sebring" in mid-March. Pete and I had been to this race once before, many years ago. The track is in the middle of nowhere. The closest hotel Pete and I could find was in a little town about forty-five minutes away. We got to the hotel the night before the race and drove to Sebring early in the morning. Michael and Jen met us at the track, driving in from Orlando after visiting with Jen's parents. Michael had found a hotel right near the track, and he got us a room at the same place. Thanks to him, we didn't have to make the long drive back to ours.

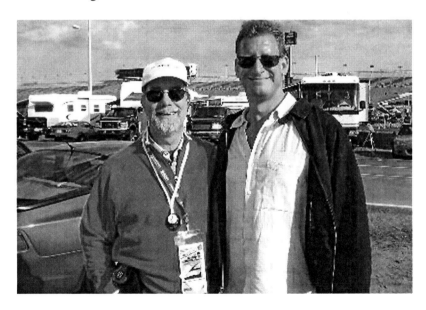

Pete and Michael at Sebring Racetrack

The race at Sebring in March was part of the American Le Mans series of racing, and was twelve hours long. It started at 10:45 a.m. that year, on March 17. Race day had brilliant blue sky and sun, although the air was cool. Pete and I both wore jackets. We found a parking place right next to the track, which gave Pete peace of mind and a place to nap. We walked the infield track like veterans, and managed the crowds and all the jostling with no problems. Jen and Michael were just fun to be with.

After the race, which Audi won, we went to dinner at a place Michael had discovered years before. The restaurant hosted a big alligator in the back courtyard. Pete was beaming. He was so happy to be sharing this event with Michael, who was the happiest we had ever seen him. It was a down-home country place with good food and a band. Pete and I danced. He was with his son, had watched race cars all day long and now had his girl by his side. Ah, that's close to heaven!

We left Michael and Jen as they returned home to the Clearwater area. Pete and I headed to Sarasota to watch a Reds spring training game at Ed Smith Stadium. The Atlanta Braves beat us badly, but Pete and I had a good time. We loved how close we were to the field. Pete and I were sitting in the sun, and for Ohioans in March, nothing else really mattered.

Pete's Carepage: March 29, 2007 @ 9:17 p.m.

Spring has arrived in Cincinnati and we are bursting with hope and thanksgiving today! Mary Jo (sister) and Pete and I went to the Cincinnati doc to get the results of the MRI. The increase in steroids did their "magic," and the injured area has shrunk significantly since the last scan. Tumors (cancer cells) don't shrink from treatment by steroids. So once again it looks like Pete's brain is still injured (inflamed) from something that no one is really sure as to the reason—but it isn't acting at all like cancer or a tumor! The "spot" which was a worry five weeks ago could hardly be seen in this month's scan.

Pete burst into a grin! Mary Jo and I shared a "high five" and the doc cautioned us that we still need to be concerned about the injured area. (Pete had just tried to "work" the doc to move his next MRI to 60 days instead of 30 days with no luck—but he did get a smile out of the doc!) But as the doc left the examining room, all three of us linked our hands and gave thanks to God for "showing up" once again and glorifying himself through his healing of Pete!

Pete's message tonight is this: "Tell them how much I appreciate their involvement. Tell them how much I appreciate their continued interest in me, and I thank them for their encouragement. And tell them I thank them most of all for their prayers." Pete asked me to tell you he is getting more involved in Crossroads (our church), and that he will find a way to give some of the good things he has received to others. Pete is grinning a lot today. And so am I. Whoo-hoo!

P.S. We had a great trip to Sebring, Florida, to see the 12 Hours of Sebring Le Mans series sports car race. Audi won. And Porsche lost to Corvette in the GT3 class (sad moment for us). The best part was spending time with son Mike and Jen, and enjoying 70 degree perfectly clear weather. After lots of visits with family and friends in Atlanta, Florida and South Carolina we made it safely home after putting over twenty-five hundred miles on the "station wagon."

P.P.S. Pete and I both "get" the HUGE impact your prayers and love and support have in continuing the positive outcomes of Pete's healing. YOU lift us up. YOU intercede for us in ways we could never do ourselves. YOUR faith and belief and RELENTLESS asking influence God's actions in our lives. How blessed we are to have every one of you!

P.P.P.S. Pete did manage to get his next MRI "pushed out" to six weeks-next MRI picture will be the second week of May. AND the doc will try lowering his steroids now to see the effect in those areas.

May your prayers continue. How we thank God for you!

§ § § § §

What a Testimony!
Patricia Ramsey April 02, 2007 at 11:03 AM EDT

God is using you, Pete, and your family to show the world what God can do through prayer. Through the love and care shared between you, your family and friends, you guys have touched more folks than any of us could have done in the last several months. Through the difficult times and the better times you have shown us how to get through it the right way—with prayer and love. Thank you, and we will continue to uplift you all in prayer because prayer does work!!!

Pat and Ron Ramsey

Congratulations on the great news!
Suzanne Fairlie April 01, 2007 at 8:40 p.m.

Pete, your story is such an inspiration to so
many others facing challenges—you and your family's
ongoing strength and prayers, and ongoing travels
to keep living life to the fullest! Hope to see you
at a pinnacle meeting in the near future, warm
regards, and continued prayers! Suzanne Fairlie.

§ § § § §

During our trip, Pete and I wrote out our goals for the year. We had
done this for years as a part of our annual New Year's routine,
although this year we were a little late. I wrote out the categories;
Pete's words are exactly as he wrote them. This man had things he
wanted to do, and as I look back on this list, brain tumor or not, he got
it done. How amazing. We went to France, not to England, but then
Pete wasn't too good with naming those things that had capital letters,
and he probably meant France instead of England when he wrote it.

GOALS—2007

Financial:	Pay our mortgage
	Will Mike & Steve
	Diversify vs. US Bank stock
Spiritual:	Relationship with God
Physical:	5 days. Eat less breakfast. Exercise. Daily Healing Touch.
	Pete eye doctor
	3 days Kathy
Mental:	Keep sharp?
Family:	Calendar identify monthly
	Weekly Mike & Steve & family
	See Mom & Dad 2 weeks
Friends:	Mike & Mary Jo Nan & Bill Pam & Mike Craig & Barbara Jack & Judith Jerry & Rose Robin Missy & Steve Judith
Church:	Volunteer. Maintain.
Community:	YWCA. United Way. Schools. Hillside Trust
Work:	Strive sale TAG (The Angus Group)
	Finalize Retirement KBN
Vacation:	Napa, Glacier, England,

Did I say Pete meant to write France instead of England? He must have, because on his list of desired things to do was the endurance race of all races in the world: The 24 Heures du Mans. Le Mans is the source of the Le Mans race car series. It is, in most opinions, the most famous sports car race in the world. It always occurs in June.

Le Mans is a little village in France, about a two-and-a-half-hour drive from Paris. Pete had watched the *24 Hours of Le Mans* race on TV for years. In fact, it was the primary reason he got the Speed channel in our cable package. The time difference made this race on TV start early on a Saturday morning in Ohio, while it was three p.m. in Le Mans. Pete even sacrificed his own prime boating time to watch this race each year.

Our trip to Le Mans began sometime in February, when Pete was reading his Porsche Club magazine, and found an advertisement for a guided tour to the race in Le Mans conducted by a travel agent located in Florida. That year was the seventy-fifth anniversary of the *24 Heures Du Mans.* Pete called for details, and found out the price and what the package included. It was very expensive. Both of us had decided that if we went, we'd invite the kids to join us—Kathy and Steve and Michael. That made it triply expensive.

I was not excited about the idea of doing a tour package. I didn't like the price. I liked the thought of going to Le Mans, but not the packaged way. Steve had gone to this race when he was a high school student on a European summer trip. We called him and he explained how massive the track was.

"It's almost ten miles long," Steve said, "and there isn't any easy way to get there." He described the village of Le Mans as a European backwater, meaning there were not many European hotels—let alone Westernized ones. "Le Mans is not on a direct route to anywhere and not near any large city," Steve informed us. "No, staying in Paris and traveling to the race is not an option," Steve said, laughing.

I started reconsidering the tour idea. Traveling in a foreign country with a husband who was ill, to a race that we had never been to before, and situated far from urban amenities, began to sound crazy if we tried to do it alone. Pete was silent as I agonized. "Let's at least get the information sent to us," I said. And we did.

The information came in boxes. We started to get excited. If we went on the packaged tour, we'd be part of a race team. We'd have access to the garage of "our" car, and special privileges in a VIP tent. All our meals during the race would be served in the tent with a gourmet French menu and wine, and on china! We'd have access to all of the garages of all of the cars. We'd be staying in a castle-type chateau in the country outside of Le Mans, and be shuttled back and forth to the race.

"Yes, they would make a special trip back to our hotel if Pete tired and needed to rest," the travel agent said.

And we would be led on our tour by Robin, a former British race car driver. He had driven the *24 Heures du Mans* a number of times. The package included a ride the day before on the track with Robin, who would give us his own personal remembrances of each turn and straightway. During the race we would be taken up into a helicopter to get a view of the racetrack like no other, and a trip to one of the curves that was remote from the rest of the fans and grandstands. Wow! Maybe it wasn't too expensive after all. This would be a trip of a lifetime. Such extravagance! How wonderful were the gifts from God! More than we had ever dreamed.

As soon as we decided to go, family and friends raised lots of caution flags. We heard on more than one occasion, "You mean you are going to travel with Pete outside of the country? What if something happens to him in France? What would you do?"

Pete and I didn't flinch. It didn't even make our worry list. We probably should have been more cautious, but we weren't. Neither of us felt any anxiety even as, at the direction of Mary Jo and Paula, we took copies of Pete's latest MRI, enough medication to survive a month and a special international phone number for the Cleveland Clinic, just in case.

The weeks before our trip had been challenging. My father ended up back in the hospital in early May after a fall in his bedroom. The doctors determined that his cancer had spread to the bones in his back, hip, pelvis, shoulders and ribs. Pete and I visited him each day as before. Dad was in tremendous pain, though alert, with lots of life in his blue eyes. Pete and Dad continued to count yellow cars in the parking lot, and talk of the Cincinnati Reds baseball team.

Dr. Albright decided he wanted to change treatment for Pete. The latest MRI showed the enhancement had grown larger as Pete's steroids were decreased. Dr. Barnett at the clinic saw that the enhancement was getting larger, too, and wanted Pete to have a biopsy performed. Dr. Barnett called and made his recommendation. I upset Pete by calling Paula back. She had called me while I was on the phone with the clinic. I told Paula the clinic's recommendation before I shared the information with Pete.

"Stop talking! Hang up!" Pete had screamed at me. "It's just you and me, baby," he said, his eyes filling with tears. "Just you and me. We need to talk and decide what to do first! I want every day I can get to be with you. I want my feet to stop swelling and my belly to stop being fat. Can you change this? What can we do to get that done?" he cried in desperation.

I hugged him, tears in my eyes too. "I'm so sorry, Pete," I said as we held each other. "Please forgive me."

"I don't want to do anything that will interfere with our trip to France and Le Mans," Pete said. "With the Cincinnati and Cleveland doctors saying biopsy, we should probably do it. I'm eighty percent there, but I don't want to make that decision today."

I was so mad at myself for not putting Pete first. How stupid of me.

Pete didn't even want to consider getting a biopsy until after our trip. But he did agree to make a visit to the clinic to learn more about the biopsy, and get a sense of the risks. I scheduled a visit to the clinic for Monday, June 4. We were leaving for Le Mans on June 12.

On Friday, June 1, my father was moved to hospice. He was in a coma-like state. My brother Joe had flown in from Oregon, and he stayed with Dad through the nights. Pete started complaining of headaches with sharp pain. His hands and feet were tingling, he said. I worried about a stroke. Dr. Albright increased Pete's steroid dosage after I called him. The headaches eased but Pete complained of vision problems, seeing "fuzzies," green stars and horses. He kept himself from driving. Pete said to me, "We might have to cancel our trip to Le Mans."

On Sunday, June 3· at two-thirty in the morning, my father died. Joe was with him. All his children and grandchildren had started a log days before. The log was near his bedside and as they visited, they would record their memories of our dad, their grandfather. It was a happy log. Whoever read it just smiled.

"You couldn't leave a better legacy than that, Dad," I whispered to him.

The next day, Pete and I, along with Mike and Mary Jo, kept our appointment at the Cleveland Clinic. Dad wouldn't have wanted Pete to miss that appointment. I was honored when Mom asked me to deliver the eulogy for my dad at his funeral on June 7.

At the clinic, Dr. Barnett did not recommend a biopsy just then. He said to continue with the increased steroid dosage, and if the enhancement got worse, assume that the tumor was back and start treating with the chemotherapy Dr. Albright recommended. If it was better, then we could back off the increased steroids.

He said the steroid taper was making it harder to interpret the MRI. "The decrease in steroids makes the change more pronounced. The inflammation is worse and the enhancement larger," Dr. Barnett told us. "But I agree with Dr. Albright, it still looks like an injury pattern, not a tumor recurrence. Enjoy Le Mans," he said. "Call this international number here at the clinic, if you have any problems. I'll be available to you."

Michael and Steven met us at our hotel in Paris on Thursday, June 14. Pete and I went over a couple of days earlier to recover from the plane ride and time change, as well as to spend a little time in Paris. We visited Sacre Coeur in the rain, and had dinner at a French street café. Pete slowly walked up all those steps at Sacre Coeur, making the handrail his best friend. Pete handled the plane ride just fine, getting up and walking in the aisles every few hours to keep his ankles from swelling more. Both of us were surprised by the Charles de Gaulle airport. We had never flown into Paris before. Our last trip to Paris had been by train from Belgium. The airport was huge! We didn't know where we were going, and I feared making Pete walk extra miles because I had guessed wrong at a turn. There was not a handrail or wheelchair in sight. We walked and we walked our way to the taxi stands. Thank goodness, I only got us lost once. Pete lugged his own bag the whole time.

Richard, our host and tour guide, picked up the four of us in Paris. He did this as a freelance job because he was a friend of Robin's. He was half French and half English. Luckily for us, we were his only pickup that day.

"This is Michael's first visit to Paris. Pete and I have only seen a few things in the city," I said to Richard. "Are we on a tight time frame? Could you give us a little driving tour of the city before we head to Le Mans?"

Richard was most gracious. He enthusiastically said yes. He gave us a native son's view of this wonderful city, highlighting the American monuments and history. He drove us around the Arc d'Triomphe, down the Champs-Elysees, by the Eiffel Tower and the Trocadero. He gave us a driving historical commentary including his own birthplace and school. He highlighted all the ways that America's history was entwined with French history, making sure we didn't miss the smaller version of our Statue of Liberty. He drove through the crazy traffic and our necks stretched this way and that, not to miss the Cathedral of

Notre Dame or the Ile of St. Louis or the window of the room where Marie Antoinette had lived her last days. How special that was. I fell in love with Paris through Richard's eyes.

Le Mans was a quaint village, beautiful in its own way. The chateau we stayed in was an old manor house. A French couple was our hosts and chefs. They showed off their talents on the evening after the race was over, serving us a seven-course traditional French dinner. From the front porch of the chateau, I could hear both the cows and the race cars in the distance at night. There were thirteen of us in the group. I was one of three women. We all had race shirts and hats for each day, emblazoned with the Le Mans logo and the name of our race team, Barazi Epsilon. The classic Gulf racing blue and orange was the color of our car. Our tickets, garage passes and pit walk passes hung proudly around our necks on lariats. We had a little strut in our walk.

On the Friday before the race, there was a parade in the village square. The cars drove down the narrow cobblestone streets while bands played and high school girls danced and cheered. The cars were the heroes to the villagers. This parade was part of the Le Mans tradition, provided for the neighbors who could not afford to go to the race. We watched the parade from a café where the windows opened out over the street. Here in a little village in France sat a couple of Americans, a Scot, some Britons, a Swede and an Australian. I had a sense of our common humanity, more alike than different. Yet in this historical place, each person represented a very different perspective on their country's history, and their view of the history of each of the countries represented by each of us around the table. I was thinking, *This must be how God's kingdom is.*

Dinner was at the Le Mans Legend on the plaza in the center of town. We were told this restaurant was a favorite of the race team. We were still eating at midnight. Pete was tiring. Earlier that day, Robin had taken us on our drive around the track. He showed us where his friend had been killed, and where he had wrecked the following year. I'll never forget him telling us that when racing down the straightway, his biggest fear was that he'd sneeze. "I couldn't risk even a second of lost concentration," he explained. "The speeds are breathtaking."

It rained the day of the race, but the showers were spotty. I was thankful for having booked the trip the way we did. A tent was set up for the race team and guests, so we did not get soaked. Richard was very kind to Pete, looking out for him and easing his way. There were no handrails anywhere at the track so we walked slowly, and carefully picked our way through the crowds.

Richard invited Michael and Steve to "protect" the Tropicana girls by holding a restraining rope against the crowds. Michael and Steve were gone in an instant to do their duty! They must have showed those pictures a hundred times: Mike and Steve, gallant soldiers, protecting the scantily dressed beauties.

We watched the pageantry of the start of the race from our seats in the grandstands after touring all the garages. It was magnificent. We had ear radios so we could hear the race in English. The colors. The music. I closed my eyes and imagined what it was like seventy-five years ago, when the drivers would physically run to their cars for the start from the opposite side of the track. Now brightly colored cars lined up in twos, one on each side, and began the race of all races.

Huge screens were strategically placed around the track so we could watch the cars maneuver their way around the 8.47-mile track. Closed circuit TVs were also in the tent and Pete spent a lot of time there, grazing on the food and wine and watching the race. As promised, we had a helicopter ride to view the track from the air. *Magnifique!* And we spent some time on a remote turn where the cars were coming off the Mulsanne Straight. A car coincidentally died near where we were, so we got a close-up view of the driver as his team radioed him fix-it instructions from the pits. Fantastic experience. Audi won. Our car, which ran in the lead position for its class through most of Saturday, crashed late Sunday morning as they pulled out of the pits. Dejection surrounded us in the garage and the tent.

Michael went home the next morning after the race while Steve, Pete and I rented a car and drove toward Normandy. We followed the country roads, N 158 out of Le Mans into Caen. We then took the D 515 north to Ouistreham and headed west, following the shoreline and the famous beaches. Pete loved World War II. He had read and studied and watched every possible movie on the war. I'd say the names of the cities out loud as we drove, and Pete nodded in recognition. Sword Beach was the first and it belonged to the British; Juno Beach to the Canadians; Gold Beach another British beachhead; then Omaha Beach and Utah Beach—the Americans!

We got out and walked Omaha Beach in silence, all of us listening for the cries of death. There was only the sound of children and families playing near the water. We walked from the beach to the slight hill above, and imagined how disadvantaged our troops were as they crawled up the sand while the German guns were blasting away at the top. A monument to the First Infantry Division, with the names of the hundreds of men killed that first day, brought a respectful reverence. Each of us walked away from the other, lost in prayer and thought and thankfulness for those who gave their lives there that day. Sacred ground still.

We stopped at the Arromanches, the artificial harbor set up by the British to ease getting equipment unloaded on to land for the offensive. There were still remnants of that harbor in the water. And we bowed to the "Rangers" as we walked through the bunkers of Point du Hoc and Pete told me the story of the courageous men who stormed that German stronghold set high above the beach at the furthest point of land stretching into the sea.

Steve had been told, after we visited the American cemetery where ten thousand Americans were buried, to make the short drive to the German cemetery where over twenty thousand German soldiers were buried. The contrast was extreme. The American cemetery was beautiful. It was a proud and patriotic place. I still remember the chills in my body as I walked from the museum to the American cemetery through a marble breezeway and heard the names of the individual soldiers buried there, being read aloud.

The German cemetery was hardly marked. No names on the grave markers; in fact, few markers placed at all. Compared to the neatly manicured American grave sites, the German graves were maintained by volunteers and showed some wear. By the evening we were back at the Charles de Gaulle Airport Hilton and had a late dinner. Pete had endured a long day. He was touched by the experience and very enthusiastic. He had liked our trip to Normandy even better than the race. Tears were in both of our eyes as we said goodbye to Steve. His traveling with us to Normandy was a special gift to both of us.

Pete's Carepage: June 28, 2007 @ 02:11 PM EDT

Pete and I have been overwhelmed by the outpouring of prayers and support for us through my father's death and our trip to Le Mans. You are wonderful friends and supporters, and your prayers keep making GREAT things happen. This is a picture of Pete and his two sons—Mike and Steve in the hospitality tent of "our" race team at Le Mans. Our trip was fabulous, truly a once-in-a-lifetime experience. Pete was safe. He did great. You would have all been proud of him, managing through the crowds of three hundred and fifty thousand at the race, climbing stairs and hills with no railings, and moving right

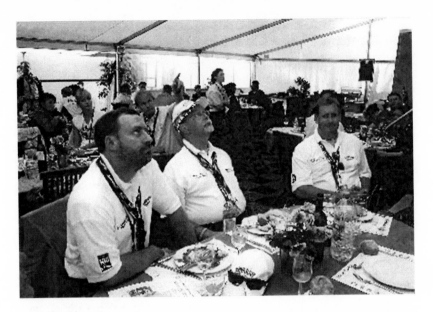

Steve, Pete, and Michael at LeMans

through his word-finding challenges even when ordering at a French restaurant off a French menu. At Le Mans, we got into the pits and the paddock, and enjoyed a helicopter ride to get a full view of the track during the race. The day before the race began, our host, a former Le Mans driver, gave us a ride on the eight-and-a-half-mile track—the famous "Mulsanne straight," "Porsche curves" and "Indianapolis turn," sharing his stories of what it was like to drive a Kremer Porsche at 230 mph. And as fantastic as the race was, Pete said his favorite part of the trip was our visit the next day to Normandy, where you could close your eyes and imagine the history playing out before you on Omaha beach. Somewhat of a religious experience!

Even MORE GOOD NEWS was our doctor visit today with the follow-up MRI. The increased steroids decreased the injured area in Pete's brain—SIGNIFICANTLY! Pete let out a whoo-hoo! No sign of a tumor. And you know it's a really good visit when the doc spends most of the visit talking about his trip to Yellowstone—giving us "tips" on how to get the best view of the animals we'll see when we head out for Glacier/Yellowstone and the Grand Tetons July 9. As soon as the doc left the room, Mary Jo and Mike (sister and brother-in-law) and Pete and me gathered hands and gave thanks and praise to God. We gave thanks for all of you and the prayers that have continued to guard Pete from harm—during our trip to France and in the healing of this injured area. HUGE relief. HUGE thanks. We are so blessed.

Pete will continue with the steroid treatment and we will take another MRI in thirty more days. "On to Glacier," Pete says with a high-five!

From my prayer journal: June 20, 2007

Thank you, Lord, for protecting Pete and me during our trip. How can I thank You enough? It was a once-in-a-lifetime experience. It was lavish. It was extravagant. How abundant are your gifts.

I remember how you taught us about extravagance. About Mary of Bethany, who had anticipated your death, and she poured a whole bottle of very expensive perfume on your head and body and wiped it with her hair. She was the only one that night that understood what you were going to be going through. I remember the disciples' criticism: This is worth more than a whole year's wages and could have been spent on the poor! And how you rebuked them. She has done a beautiful thing, you said. And then you said that whenever your story would be told, you wanted her story to be included. That is the only time you said that. How nice of you to make sure her story was included. And how nice you are to allow Pete to experience some of this same kind of extravagance as he gets ready to go through what he will have to go through. No other God but you would think of that!

17

Finishing the Dream Trip

We got back from Le Mans and spent some time on our boat. I watched Pete struggle to get up and down the steps to the bridge of the boat. I watched him struggle to get up and down from the floor. How his hands and arms shook when he tried to help me snap the canvas down! I got alarmed when he told me he didn't remember which switches to turn off when we left the boat, because I didn't know either. But then, it was Pete who remembered we needed to check the switches at all, not me.

These changes made me think Pete was getting worse. His balance was more of a challenge for him, and his walk less steady than it had been. He seemed more confused to me, like when he couldn't remember where we kept the barbeque sauce in the kitchen. But then he would surprise me and smoke his ribs, making not just one type of sauce but three sauces—all wonderful and all different. How he loved doing his ribs in the smoker!

Such a strange mix of feelings. I had flashbacks of what Pete used to be able to do, and I felt so sad. I mourned the loss of that man, and at the very same time, admired more than ever the man he had become. He was much more direct with his feelings and desires. So much more transparent. He laughed more than ever. He appreciated the small things, and always gave thanks. I think I respected him now for different things. For his courage to have faced his illness and fight through it. I admired his childlike trust in God. His appreciation for every day. His desire to keep walking and doing things. His desire for Le Mans. His drive to make Montana happen. His refusal to just sit. His willingness to continue to meet new people. His loyalty to his school boards and his CEO Roundtable. His desire to support the business of the Angus group. His faithfulness to spending time with my mother who was now grieving. He kept driving. He still made good decisions and had good judgment. I trusted him. And, as always, he counseled me. And was usually right.

He told me that he hated it when I asked him how he was doing. He hated it when I tried to encourage him about how well he was doing. He hated it when I pointed out any of his differences from the way he was before. He saw that as a sign of weakness and fought it.

It must have felt like a lack of respect for him when I did this. So I stopped.

Pete was motivated by trips. We had made it to Le Mans. We had visited Mount Rushmore, and made it salmon fishing. The rest of the trip, we had originally planned, was to visit Yellowstone and the Tetons.

In talking to Nan and Bill, they convinced us to include Glacier Park in Montana as part of our trip. In fact, we invited them to go with us. They had been the year before, and longed to go back. They knew where we should stay and what to see. They had no interest in heading to Yellowstone or the Tetons, so after Glacier they would head north to Canada. Pete and I convinced Mary Jo and Mike to join us also. They had never been to Yellowstone or the Tetons, and had those destinations on their list, too.

I was probably more excited about this trip than Le Mans. Pete got a bad cold right before we left, and for a few days the trip was at risk. But we stayed positive. Nan checked the status of the roads in Glacier daily. She'd report to all of us. The snow finally melted shortly after July 4. The "Going to the Sun" road was now open, and was the must-do for the Glacier trip. It is one of the world's most spectacular highways. It is fifty miles long, cutting through the heart of Glacier, hugging the cliffs, crossing the Continental Divide and Logan's Pass in the Rocky Mountains. The six of us left for Montana on July 9.

Glacier National Park was not the easiest place to get to. We flew into Salt Lake City from Cincinnati, then hopped a regional flight from Salt Lake to Kalispell, Montana, and drove from Kalispell along the southern border of Glacier National Park for several hours to get to the Glacier Park Lodge. Nan met us at the lodge so distressed. She was worried that their choice for accommodations would disappoint us.

"We can move. We don't have to stay here," Nan said. "Bill and I haven't unpacked yet, just in case you want to move."

Nan and Bill had gotten to the lodge a few hours ahead of us, catching an earlier flight to Kalispell. The four of us laughed! Nan was a perfectionist in her dress and her home. She had a high standard, and she was so worried about offending us. This was the first time we had traveled together. This park lodge was, shall we say, a little rustic. All Pete cared about was getting a room on the first floor so he could avoid the steps. And that we did! The lodge was fine. In fact, the grounds were gorgeous with all the spring wildflowers in bloom. The lobby was built with huge redwood trees that made the ceiling tower above us. It was an unforgettable kind of place.

Pete developed a real sensitivity to any kind of wind in his eyes during this trip. He would close them regularly, and avoid any place where the wind was blowing. Since we were in the mountains, blowing wind happened a lot. The doctor later said that sensitivity was an effect of the steroids. This made Glacier a challenging experience for Pete, coupled with his inability to walk long distances. His favorite thing amidst all this beauty was seeing the long-horned sheep at Logan's Pass, and discovering a bear near the road near St. Mary's Lake. He never complained, but his lack of enthusiasm was evident.

One afternoon, I got Pete fishing while the others went hiking. I hired a guide who took us out to a very remote lake on the Indian reservation next to the park. Ranchers on horseback herding their cattle were the only civilization we saw all day. Our guide was a dear man, and he was especially kind to Pete. We put on our waders, and were ready to launch our rowboat when Pete announced he'd stay in the truck while I went fishing. The wind coming down off the mountains across the plains hurt his eyes too much. Finally Pete got into the boat when the wind died down after watching me fish for an hour or so. We didn't catch anything that day.

There was a sacred spot called Running Eagle Falls in Glacier National Park that Bill had discovered during his last trip. Running Eagle was a great woman warrior of the Blackfoot people. She found her strength and power during her meditations at the falls. There she received her medicine and healing. This power made her a great leader. Bill did healing touch on Pete while we were at the Running Eagle Falls, aligning himself and Pete with the energy of this great woman warrior. Bill said the falls was a site of an energy vortex in the earth, which was why it was so powerful in its healing.

From Montana, we headed south into Wyoming through Yellowstone and found a wonderful spot to stay at Jackson Lake Lodge in the Tetons. Elk grazed in the back valley just beyond the lodge patio. The majestic Tetons rose above the valley. Bailey's Irish Cream on the patio with a full moon made us all smile. Pete's enthusiasm returned. In fact, he was ecstatic as we chased wildlife through the Tetons and Yellowstone. They were living in abundance in both parks. We saw lots of elk, and chased a bull elk one afternoon near the glorious Tower Falls in Yellowstone. We found a moose grazing near a creek on a very remote road in the Tetons, and later that night chased another moose and her calf up the road from where we were staying. The chase would end when we had exhausted our digital cameras. We saw osprey, hundreds of buffalo, plenty of white-tailed deer and Pete's favorite—bears! The drought that summer had driven the bears further down out of the mountains in Yellowstone in their search for food. We were the lucky beneficiaries. There was Pete, who struggled to walk, scrambling out of the back seat of the car, and walking and walking and walking for a view of those big black creatures lumbering along. How delighted he was! Many big black bears roamed the hillsides. Some got so close the rangers yelled at us. In the early hours of the evening after dinner, we'd drive to a pond and spend the last hours of sunlight watching beavers and otters play in the pond with the egrets and swans.

We spent hours driving and looking. Pete was like a kid. We all were. How fun it was. The geysers, springs, mud pots, lakes, waterfalls and mountains wowed Mary Jo and me, but Mike and Pete were like hunters seeking glimpses of animals day and night. They were not disappointed. For Pete, seeing all this wildlife was worth all the travel time—and the wind that irritated his eyes. His enthusiasm for the animals gave him the courage to keep up the effort to walk. This was close to heaven!

Mike, Mary Jo and me commented how lucky we were to be traveling with Pete. It was like God gave him special favors. Since we were with him, we got the benefit. Picking good spots to stay and to eat in places we had never been before. We always got the best seating at restaurants, near the windows. It never rained. Pete didn't get sick the whole trip. There were always rooms available on the first floor. And the animals! God's gift to Pete!

Pete's Carepage: August 8, 2007 @ 6:35 p.m.

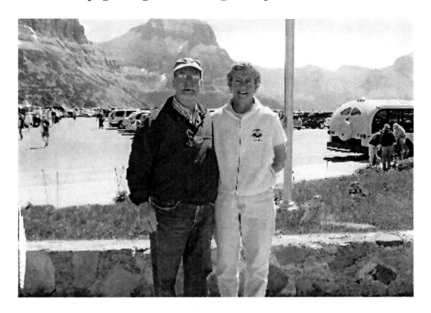

The picture says it all: Pete and I at Logan's Pass in Glacier National Park in Montana. Thanks to each of you who prayed us there and back. We were safe and we had a BLAST! We spent half of our time at the Lodge in Glacier and half the time at Jackson Lake Lodge in the Tetons visiting Yellowstone from there. The beauty was incredible. The geology fascinating. Sister Mary Jo and Mike, and our healers Bill and Nan, joined us on this trip.

Pete says (as I write) the trip was a lot of fun! We just didn't get to see "big" land but also all the people who were so engaged in all the park activities. I liked the animals the best! We saw so many, and so many different kinds and we got so close to them—even got to chase a few. We saw an eagle, osprey, buffalo, elk, a moose and her calf, beaver, otters, pronghorn, mule deer, big horn sheep, and even two black bears!

Pete got the next set of MRIs done last week, and both Cincinnati and Cleveland Clinic docs were pleased that the steroids were containing the injured area and maybe was even slightly better. GREAT news! The bad news is the toll the steroids are having on Pete. He has difficulty walking any kind of distance; his balance is shaky; his weight is the highest ever; his arms bleed; his ankles are swollen; and his reading and writing have regressed. But as Pete says, "I'm doing

GREAT day-to-day. I don't have a bad day (and neither do I). Every morning I wake up and give thanks to God that I am alive and I have another day." Pete never complains about the side effects except he hates "being fat."

So we can't thank you enough for your continued belief in us, love for us and prayers for us. It's been over eighteen months since diagnosis. Your prayers make a difference. We can feel the lift and it is awesome.

Pray now for the docs and Pete and my wisdom in discovering the next step for treatment for Pete. There is a lot of discussion (but not many options) about steroids alternatives. THANK YOU! THANK YOU!

From my prayer journal: July 18, 2007

Your peace this morning takes away the sadness I have felt this whole trip. I see Pete's capabilities decreasing. Mary Jo and Mike both confirmed how much worse he is since January's trip with them to Daytona. Less stamina, endurance, balance and memory. It makes me sad and makes it real to me. Pete seems unaware and not frustrated at all. I am sad because it means, Lord, that you are not healing Pete. I know you don't heal marginally—you'd bring Pete to full recovery or not at all. All the signs say you are not going to heal him. But I know you are with us. I don't fear being abandoned by you. I get afraid of a long and debilitating time ahead with Pete. I feel fear and hopelessness. And then I remember what you have done already! Pete is now at nineteen months of living! His life expectancy had been for six to eleven months. No tumor has recurred. He is able to walk and talk and still has his spirit! Ah! Yes I appreciate your grace. You are good. You give Pete and me your presence and your grace. I entrust Pete to you. I believed you when you said, "Don't let your hearts be troubled. I am with you." And I will not lose hope! Your time is not our time. I will keep asking you relentlessly for Pete's full and complete healing. I'll keep expecting miracles from you and simultaneously accepting that you may chose not to. Either way, your promise is to stay with us. And your presence is enough.

18

Living with Uncertainty

The diagnosis of Pete's brain tumor was pretty certain. Early on, all the doctors agreed it looked and acted like a glioblastoma multiforme brain tumor. The tumor's aggressiveness gave it a Grade IV rating. The pathology reports after Pete's surgery confirmed what they thought. Although we felt anxiety about the surgery and the clinical trial, little did we know that we had just finished the most certain leg of our journey. From now on we were traveling in shades of grey and uncertainty.

Once the tumor was removed, the attention of the doctors and medical staff was on Pete's functionality and the possible recurrence of the tumor. The doctors' ability to determine what was going on in Pete's brain was dependent on tests, primarily the MRI, and any symptoms Pete might have that could give them clues. But the ability to interpret the MRI was not an exact science. Our doctors had looked at thousands of MRIs over the years they practiced. Each time Pete got a new MRI, the tumor boards of each hospital reviewed it, so we had the collective experience of many experts. But they still were never absolutely certain of what they saw.

I was initially surprised that the doctors couldn't tell for sure what was going on in Pete's brain. For awhile, I kept thinking they would be able to. But it slowly dawned on me and Pete: they couldn't. It was not a question of competence, but a statement about the tools and tests currently available to them. Neurological treatment and diagnosis had advanced very far in the last twenty years, but the tests still couldn't make fine enough distinctions. Was the white haze on the MRI the tumor recurring? Or was it dead tissue as a result of treatment? Uncertainty was a condition that just was.

The next four Carepage updates demonstrated the roller-coaster ride of uncertainty over a five-week period of time in 2006. This ride took place seven months from tumor removal surgery; five months from pneumonia; four months from blood clots and one month after Pete passed his driving test!

Pete's Carepage: August 14, 2006 @ 9:58 p.m.

Okay, it's time for some heightened levels of prayer! Pete's latest MRI does not look clean. There is something that is showing up, and both our Cincinnati doc and the Cleveland Clinic indicate that there is a good chance it is tumor activity. Over the next week, more tests are required and then once it gets a little clearer, we will need to make some decisions about treatment options.

Pete and I are obviously disappointed. We are asking God where He is taking us next on this journey. We turn our fears over to Him and trust his continuing presence with us and His purposes. I am reminding Him to continue His healing work in Pete—he doesn't leave His work half-finished!

On a lighter note, Pete continues to do very well. He made six miles on his bike Saturday, a new mileage milestone, all signs of his continued strength improvement. And we have gone back to our volunteer role at Crossroads church. We worked the Info Center the last two weekends and Pete answered member questions readily. How warmly we were greeted on our return! Thank you, Crossroads members!

I have learned that we need to pray for specifics, so here is my request. Have I told you lately how much we count on the power of your prayer? Join us in being bold in asking God to kill all the cancer cells in Pete's brain. We know we are in a battle, and we need all the power of prayer in this battle. Ask God to also give Pete and me wisdom in making decisions about his treatment. Thank you so much for your faithfulness to us over all these months. We knew this journey would be a long one, and you have been persevering in your following of us.

A short week later, the news got worse. Chemotherapy was scheduled as soon as we returned from Mount Rushmore.

Pete's Carepage: August 21, 2006 @ 10:08 p.m. EDT

Thanks to all for your unbelievable response to Pete and I. God has to be sick of hearing from you about us! You are a wonderful army to have—so "fierce" in your praying. Pete and I are grateful for how you lift us.

Quick update: Pete had a specialized MRI called a spectroscopy last week. It measures the chemical make-up of the cells so a determination can be made about what is going on. We met with the doctor and he told us the test was not "diagnostic," meaning he can't draw any definitive conclusions from it. He knows there is damage being done, it has some characteristics of a tumor, but he can't say definitely whether it is or not. He did say that we can't just sit and watch it. So the only other way to determine a diagnosis would be to go back to the Cleveland Clinic and have a biopsy completed—which is another surgery and has its own set of risks without any treatment "benefit" for Pete. So we have decided not to do that. Pete has come so far, he just can't even consider risking that progress. So we will be starting chemotherapy in Cincinnati under Dr. Albright's direction. BUT before we do, we are going to take a portion of that BIG trip out West while we can, and will be leaving for Mount Rushmore and the Badlands and the Black Hills tomorrow.

Please continue to storm the heavens as you have this last week, praying for an elimination of any cancer cells in Pete's brain and his overall strength to get him ready for chemo.

P.S. Our "healing touch" guy, Bill, got us connected to a Medical Intuitor (sp?), a Ph.D. doc (not an MD doc) who has been in practice for a long time and can "read" energy fields. (The nurses who works with her say she is more accurate than an MRI!) She was encouraging to us, saying she could not "see" any significant cancer in Pete's body and was more worried about his intestinal system than his brain. Go figure!

§ § § § §

YOU'RE IN GOOD HANDS!! [Rom. 8:37–39]
Peter Lamb—August 22, 2006 at 11:42 AM EDT

Hi Pete and Kathy,

   Diane and I continue to hold you up in our prayers, believing that in Christ, your Heavenly

Father is, right now, reaching to you in amazing
love and grace, to accomplish what He desires (what
He "wills") to do in your lives! Though you may be
facing a time of particular testing, don't lose
heart, for you can trust your Father, who loves
you. You are in His grip!

You're gonna have a blast out West! Enjoy the
sunsets and sunsets—they are spectacular in that
part of the country!!! Our prayers go with you.

Your Friends,
Peter and Diane Lamb

Back from Mount Rushmore—ready for chemotherapy to start.
Resigned to the fact the tumor had recurred even though Pete was
doing so well. Plan changed again!

Pete's Carepage: September 02, 2006 @ 5:08 PM EDT

*We had a great trip to Mount Rushmore and the Black Hills. To all
of our South Dakota friends: WOW—what a beautiful country. The
wildlife was especially pleasing to Pete—hundreds of buffalo, deer,
wild turkeys and other animals. The beautiful hills and Needles
helped me realize why the Indians thought the hills were sacred, and
the beauty was soothing and comforting to me. Both of us loved the
roads—two of the "best roads in America" are in the Black Hills, and
we drove each more than once! Thanks to all of you for your good
wishes and prayers for safe travels. We had a marvelous few days!*

*We had planned to start chemotherapy this past Thursday. Wednes-
day afternoon I received a call from the Cleveland Clinic and, after
looking at the spectroscopy, Dr. Barnett (and subsequently members
of their Tumor Board) thought the spectroscopy was not suggestive of
tumor. So we slowed down a little, and after visiting with our Cincinnati doc decided that we would wait and scan/test again, and that
should give us better guidance. The clinic suggested putting Pete on a
low dose of steroids to see if the area in question is some kind of
inflammation which the steroids could shrink. So—the next tests are
Sept. 19, with visits to both our Cincinnati doc and the Cleveland
Clinic to follow that week to get the best advice.*

*So—the journey continues. Perhaps God's guiding hand is on us,
and all of your prayers storming the heavens are having influence!
Thanks for helping us in the battle! Pete continues to do just great!
Here's a picture of him the first day he captained his boat!*

The testing schedule allows us to get in our salmon fishing trip to Oregon that my brother Joe promised and has so graciously arranged. We leave Sept. 11 for Oregon, and after visiting our good friends Dick and Abby in Bend, we'll meet up with my brother and family to catch some salmon (I'm optimistic) in the Columbia River! You can be sure if we are successful, pictures will adorn this Carepage!

Keep praying for the destruction of Pete's cancer cells! We count on your passion and love for us, which lifts us every day, and your faith and belief in God's powerful love.

§ § § § §

Anything is possible
Charlotte Manison August 29, 2006 at 04:55 PM EDT

I hope, when you looked at the magnificence of Mount Rushmore and the impressive forests of the Black Hills where the cathedral spires poke out of the trees, you reflected that truly, anything is possible. Between what God made and what man made in that small little piece of the Black Hills, it should comfort you to know that between God and man, cancer cells can be made to go away too. Hope you had a FABULOUS trip! I enjoyed my trip to that part of the country a few years ago very much.

§ § § § §

Hi!
Jo Ann Hopkins September 02, 2006 at 09:33 PM EDT

Hi, Pete and Kathy. What encouraging news about the chemo, or lack of it, and the possibility that there is just an infection. We will certainly be praying that way, and of course, that no cancer cells are lurking in Pete. Did you read in the paper about the gene therapy for cancer cells by training our own white cells to attack cancer cells in our body? They're going to conquer this "monster" yet!

So happy you had a nice trip. Pete sounds like a "wild turkey" himself, with all he's accomplishing! God is SO good to allow you to have the trip for salmon fishing. That is beautiful country out there, and we'll pray for traveling mercies, good weather, and a fish or two.

```
     I  am  not  able  to  come  to  the  prayer  gathering
tomorrow,  but  you  know  that  I  will  be  praying  here,
as  will  Gil.  We  are  so  blessed  to  be  able  to  share
this  journey  (or  is  it  a  "trek"?)  with  you,  and  see
how  God  continues  to  work  in  your  life,  Pete.  Our
faith  has  grown  as  we  have  witnessed  your  trust  in
the  Lord  through  all  of  this,  and  seen  how  faithful
He  is,  and  how  willing  He  is  to  "bend  low"  to  touch
our  lives.
Love,
Jo  Ann
```

As the responses to our Carepages demonstrate, the faith and support of others during Pete's and my journey helped us deal with our own uncertainty. Their encouragement helped ease my fears. Their humor and teasing of Pete made him laugh. He felt so blessed to have so many people taking an interest in him.

Pete never whined about the doctors' uncertainty. I didn't either. What right did I have to whine when he didn't? But whine to God, I did. I'd bring my fears to him on so many days—too many to count. Somehow, by sharing my fears and asking for God's guidance in all the treatment decisions Pete and I had to make, I'd find peace. Here's where I learned that fear and love can't exist simultaneously. Choose love, I'd tell myself. If I focused on Pete and his needs and wants, my fear would disappear. Choose to trust, I'd tell myself. "Keep my eyes fixed on Jesus," I would repeat day after day. "You are the Path. My only job was to follow." I trusted. "You'll lead us out of this jungle." And He did.

The spectroscopy mentioned in the Carepage update was a specialized form of an MRI. Pete went to the same place where he had gotten his previous MRIs, but instead of a twenty-minute test, the MRI/spectroscopy took almost two hours. Pete never complained about lying still that long with his head in a tin can. He never complained about the noise. The staff gave him extra blankets to keep him warm in the cold testing room. The staff talked to him to keep him awake, so they had his brain waves moving as they took pictures. They all fell in love with Pete, especially Joyce; she looked out for him and would walk him into the MRI picture room from the waiting room. Pete always smiled his wonderful smile when he saw her.

The spectroscopy actually gave us a picture graph that measured chemical reactions to the cells in Pete's brain when stimulated. Those chemical reactions were represented by different lines on a graph.

Each line on the graph measured a different chemical reaction. The ratio of choline to creatine would suggest the highest chance of a tumor; the ratio of lactate to creatine would suggest the cells were dead, and probably necrosis was present from radiation or the IL-13 treatment. Pete's MRI/Spectroscopy (MRS) almost always showed a clear injury pattern from dead scar tissue, not new tumor activity. The test was by no means one hundred percent accurate. It gave false positives frequently.

One of the real challenges in Pete's case was not knowing what we were looking at on the MRI. Was it tumor growth or scar tissue or radiation damage or damage from the IL-13 drug? It all showed up as white stuff on the MRI. The only good MRI is one with no white stuff. And Pete didn't have any of those.

Dr. Albright, during our visit with him in August of 2006, said that the spectroscopy was not diagnostic, meaning he couldn't draw any definitive conclusions from it. He did know damage was being done. It might be the tumor recurring, or it might not be a tumor at all. He said, "We can't sit and watch it. It will keep causing damage." Dr. Albright recommended starting chemotherapy right away.

Pete cried when he told Steven on the phone that August of 2006 that the doctors thought the tumor was back. He was so disappointed. His hopes were dashed. My heart broke. Pete and I prayed this prayer together that night: "Do not turn your back on Pete, Lord. Do not turn away your face. We have relied on you! Please accomplish what you have begun in Pete."

From my prayer journal: August 22, 2006

I screamed in my prayer journal. How my heart is aching! Where are you taking us now? How do I make sense of this? MRI results seem to show that the tumor is back. It looks like it is growing on the rim where the surgery was done. Does this mean that you really didn't heal Pete? We were mistaken in reading Pete's improvement as your work? You didn't really heal him? We gave praise and glory to you and it wasn't your work at all? I know you don't heal marginally. All the stories of your healing are complete. You are the God of abundance. You don't heal "kind of." Was the testimony that we gave about you false? A hope constructed only in our own minds? So many non-believers will say: "See, they thought God was with them but He's not." It will confirm in them that they are right in not believing in you. Is this a test of our faith in you?

We have put our lives in your hands. We are willing to accept your will, whatever it is, whatever your purpose is, your plan for us.

And you said to me: "My action is in you and Pete's response to this news. My presence is in your love of each other and your trust in me. The test of my presence with you is not dependent on the healing of Pete."

I recalled with hope the story in the Bible about the long journey in the desert by the Israelites. Larry Crabb, in his book *Inside Out,* put it this way. "His promise of daily bread and His pledge to supply us with what we need according to His riches must be carefully understood to mean that we can count on receiving from God all that's necessary to achieve *His purpose* in our life." [Emphasis mine] As Numbers says, God directed them so: "When the Cloud moves, you move; when the Cloud stops, you stop." Crabb goes on to picture God saying, "You will never learn to trust me until you come to terms with my authority. Trust will never emerge from a *demanding spirit* [emphasis mine]. Let's start with a clear understanding. I give the orders. You do what you are told. With that as a beginning, you will eventually taste my goodness and richness of fellowship with me and come to trust me deeply. God opposes the proud who demand, but he gives grace to the humble who express their hurt."

I became aware of my own faulty thinking. On some level, I kept thinking that my faith in God would heal Pete. If I prayed hard enough, if I gave Him enough glory, I'd get what I wanted. How silly I was. I was bargaining with God. It's not my effort or my faith. It's only God's grace and purpose that matter.

19

Living with More Uncertainty

Pete didn't want to go to the Cleveland Clinic for the biopsy. I really wanted him to go. I felt like we needed to know what we were up against, and that seemed the only way. Both docs said that the biopsy was not without risk. Bleeding was the risk, since the biopsy was a surgical procedure, and Pete's skull would have to be opened again so Dr. Barnett could withdraw some tissue. The clinic reassured us that the risk was small. But they also reminded us that we could do the biopsy, and it was possible that we still wouldn't know for sure what was going on in Pete's brain. Sometimes they couldn't get the right tissue to make a definitive call. Pete didn't want anything to do with more surgery. I understood why he didn't. But I agonized. I believed we should go, and I could not persuade Pete. He did agree to go to the clinic for an exam and assessment.

Pete was doing well. This gave him less desire to have another surgical procedure done. We went to the planning retreat for his two school boards in early August 2006 at one of our favorite places, the Griffin Gate Marriott in Lexington, Kentucky. He went to the meetings, and we went together to the social dinner. He was happy, talking with his fellow board members easily. It felt like a little mini-vacation for us.

The next day, there was Pete at the Crossroads picnic for our volunteer group. He stood for hours. Amazed me. He spoke with all present, and was so gracious and friendly. He laughed a lot. The only complaint he had was that he was having a little trouble hearing.

We visited a few new doctors to get answers to things Pete was uncertain about, and were worrying him. Pete had a colonoscopy done. He was always worried that he would die from colon cancer, which was what killed his father. Some people thought it was crazy for Pete to get a colonoscopy. Given the slow growth of colon cancer, even if he had it, the brain tumor would get him way before the colon cancer would. But Pete had anxiety about this. It was a pleasure for me to do anything for him, which would make his way easier. So we got the colonoscopy done and he was relieved to find out that his colon was just fine!

Then off we went to the ear doctor to find out about his hearing issues. The doctor said that high-pitched sounds were difficult for Pete, probably caused by some sort of trauma. The radiation may have contributed to it. Pete didn't need a hearing aid yet; we just needed to live around it by avoiding very noisy rooms.

Crossroads organized another prayer service for Pete in early September. So many friends and family members and crossroads members came. I was overwhelmed with the outpouring of love. Pete and I sat next to each other in the front of the chapel. Tears streamed down my face. Pete kept his head bowed. They anointed Pete and me with oil for healing and to give us strength.

Pete had his next MRI/Spectroscopy. Dr. Albright said that the "pictures are interesting." They definitely showed less intensity or enhancement and the spectroscopy showed a definite injury pattern versus a tumor pattern. Dr. Albright was still worried about "some kissing spots" near one of the chambers of Pete's brain. Dr. Albright knew we were off to the Cleveland Clinic the next day. He asked us to update him on our assessment after the visit. We agreed to do so.

Mary Jo and Mike went with us to the clinic. Dr. Stevens, the oncologist at the clinic, said Dr. Albright was putting a lot of weight on the spectroscopy, which was difficult to do. He believed that the tumor hadn't progressed, but he recommended a different medication for treatment.

We then met with Pete's surgeon, Dr. Barnett. Our primary reason for the visit was to determine whether we should do a biopsy or not. Dr. Barnett suddenly was not so enthusiastic about doing a biopsy. He said the area in Pete's brain definitely looked to him like an injury, not a tumor. There was definitely some inflammation there; Dr. Barnett was not sure of the cause.

"It could be a reaction from Pete's immune system to the IL-13. Who knows? The area would be difficult to get to biopsy, and Pete would have to do a lot more than just wear lime green life-saver stickers on his head," Dr. Barnett said.

Dr. Barnett would have had to use screws to get into Pete's skull. Pete's decision not to do a biopsy was the right one!

The chemotherapy that was supposed to have started before our salmon fishing trip was now not needed from both Dr. Barnett's and Dr. Albright's perspective. This was September of 2006.

I couldn't help myself. I silently sang God's praise. His handiwork seemed evident to me. He did not step away from us. And how much deeper was my belief and trust in Pete's decisions.

Pete's Carepage: September 23, 2006 @ 2:34 p.m.

Pete and I and our two faithful angels, Mary Jo and Mike, stopped for dinner on our way home from the Cleveland Clinic last night. We raised our wine glasses and toasted God with hearts full of thanks, proclaiming his glory. The prior twenty-four hours included three doctor visits. Each of them had a little different "spin" on what the latest MRI and spectroscopy told them, but all came to a consensus that it looks like the damage occurring in Pete's brain now is more of an "injury" than a tumor. Dr. B pulled the original scans taken right after Pete's surgery, and confirmed that the area showing damage now is right where he had placed one of the catheters and IL-13 drug. Both docs said that the spectroscopy rarely gives "false negatives," which in English means, you can be pretty sure if this picture says "it isn't a tumor—it ain't!" Whoo-hoo! How much of a miracle it is that these medical doctors are cooperating so well together in helping Pete! AND they are agreeing. And all the "starts-and-stops" and differences of viewpoint in the last few weeks have indeed turned out so right. So they say: "No need for chemo—no need for biopsy" and we say: "Lots of reason for rejoicing and giving thanks!" Pete says to tell everyone he's "very happy," and he thanks each of you for your fierce prayers and ongoing support. God has once again shown his faithfulness, and is completing the healing in Pete he began months ago. The clinic staff had not seen Pete since early February, when he was very sick and wheelchair bound. Pete heard the docs and staff from the clinic use words like "remarkable" and "marvelous" as they examined him and described his recovery. We know that God has indeed shown how marvelous He is in Pete, and we also know all too well how your prayers, unwavering belief and requests for Pete's healing have influenced just how remarkable He is! So join us in a little adult beverage of your choice when you read this, and make the toast of thankfulness with us.

We moved into a routine of getting the MRI/Spectroscopy (MRS) completed each month. We would have the results reviewed with a visit with Dr. Albright in Cincinnati, followed by a phone call from Dr. Barnett with his and the tumor board's assessment at the Cleveland Clinic. The damaged area in Pete's brain was still expanding, but the damage still looked convincingly like an injury rather than new tumor growth. The clinic kept prescribing the lowest level of steroids Pete could handle, and still keep the enhancement in check. Dr. Albright kept reminding us that Pete's brain tissue was still being damaged, and would cause Pete harm even though it was not a tumor. Dr. Albright would have liked to do more aggressive therapy using chemotherapy and Avastin.

Pete and I repeatedly opted for the "do nothing and enjoy the quality of life we have while we have it" option. I came to the conclusion that Pete and my future was an endless series of uncertain circumstances. I came to peace with that. I stopped asking God what was next. My only job was to focus on Pete, and do it to my very best! I felt great joy in that realization, and I loved each day.

It was the end of October, and the end of the boating season. Pete captained the boat out of our dock slip, and to the marina where it would be stored until next spring. Pete captained the boat by himself, and drove it right on to the trailer to haul it out of the water. That was not the easiest of maneuvers, fighting against a river current and wind. Pete did it perfectly.

A few days later, we finished Pete's taper of steroids. He was off of them completely now, for the first time since surgery. Almost immediately, Pete started having more difficulty with word finding. He would get frustrated. His driving and mobility were fine, but everything else seemed to be slowing down. He developed a rash on his ankles and some swelling. We put the support hose back on, since we had a big trip ahead of us.

We left for our second trip to Florida right after Pete's seven-thirty a.m. school board meeting the first of November. We drove to Atlanta that first night, Pete doing a good majority of the driving, and then on to Clearwater. Michael was as happy as we had ever seen him, living with Jen and her daughter, Chelsea. Michael was amazed at his dad.

"How well you are doing," Michael exclaimed. "Just like years ago. You are like you used to be. No different," he said, hugging his father. Pete beamed. Then Michael turned to me and said a kind thing: "He is lucky to have you."

"It's his courage, Michael," I said. My heart rejoiced at Michael's amazement.

I watched for any change in Pete with the lower steroid dosage. There was not much change at all. He seemed a little quieter than usual at the group dinners. I asked him if he was having trouble following or hearing conversations. "Both," he simply said, and did not offer any more.

I thought that Pete might be forgetting a little more. He called me from the car one day because he couldn't remember how to get to our clothes repair shop, but as soon as I gave him a landmark, he remembered instantly. On another day, he couldn't remember the name of our favorite ice cream store. He was driving all the time when we went out together, and I remember how he couldn't remember how to get to Hyde Park, a very familiar and often-visited neighborhood. On another day, he had trouble knowing how to get to the post office, which he had done a million times before. But the memory lapses weren't consistent, which was all the more maddening for me! Pete would forget how to get to the post office one day, and on the very next day, he'd get all dressed up in a suit and tie and take his colleague from the Angus group to a chamber meeting to introduce her around to all the people he knew. He had no problems getting there or back and there he was—the man who couldn't remember any names introducing his colleague to his contacts. Go figure!

Right before Christmas, Pete told me of a recurring dream he had. "I am caught in the hospital and I can't get out. It's awful. And it keeps playing over and over."

I knew Pete hated being in a hospital. We prayed that our visits would be infrequent.

Pete's January 2007 MRI showed no worsening. We felt relief as always. The Cleveland Clinic wanted Pete to get a PET scan. Dr. Albright was not as enthusiastic, because he didn't think the results of a PET scan were very reliable for brain cancer detection. However, he agreed to order the procedure. Pete and I visited a PET scan center to get the test done. Pete ended up making a friend with the technician, Jim. A week later they went to lunch. Only Pete!

PET stands for Position Emission Tomography, a type of nuclear medicine imaging. Pete got a radiotracer injected into his vein through an IV, and then Pete had to stay quiet for about forty-five minutes, waiting for the tracer to get to the right part of Pete's body. That's when he and Jim became friends. The actual time of the scan was another forty-five minutes. The clinic wanted the PET done to see if they could determine if Pete's brain cancer had returned, since the MRI was so difficult to interpret.

During the PET scan, if the radiotracer accumulated more in one part of Pete's body than another, it emitted gamma rays. Gamma rays were a small amount of energy that could be detected by a gamma camera, and gave a picture of the chemical activity in Pete's body. Cancerous cells tend to accumulate more of the radiotracer than normal cells, so if cancerous cells are present, the picture will show a "hot" spot. Pete's PET scan didn't show any "hot" spots, which was a good thing. The doctors were glad to now have a baseline PET scan, so if Pete's future MRI showed some change, they could order another PET scan to confirm what kind of change it was.

Pete's Carepage: February 22, 2007 @ 10:45 p.m.

A little bit of noise! Had our Cincinnati doctor visit today to review the MRI. It has been six weeks since we had the last MRI. We had hoped to move to eight weeks after this visit, but no such luck. The injured area that has been present in Pete's brain has gotten bigger in the last six weeks. It still does NOT look like it is tumor/cancer activity, but the injured area getting bigger is a concern. The Cincinnati doc feels like we need to change treatment, to get this injured area to stabilize or shrink. What that new treatment should be is being discussed. Conversations with the Cleveland Clinic are ongoing.

So stay posted. For now, pray for wisdom of the doctors and ask for good guidance for Pete, as we make the decisions as to what the next treatment steps should be.

Right after this doctor visit, Pete and I drove to Chicago to attend a wedding of one of his cousins. Although we did not know this cousin very well, the wedding was bringing his whole family together. The Detroit family was coming in with their families to be with us and the Chicago family. Pete, being an only child, had grown up with Char as his sister and Don as his older brother. He used to talk frequently about the good times he'd had visiting them in Detroit. Don had introduced him to older-brother things like beer, smoking, cars and girls. There was a bond between them that was strong and loving. Char had been the caring and nurturing one. How much she loved Pete. She called Pete regularly, as did Don, to check in.

The family gathering was one of the warmest, most loving times with the family we had ever had. I found out during that visit from Vi, Pete's aunt, that Pete had found his mom when she died. He had been doing his homework and heard a thud. Pete ran into the bathroom, felt her heart, and found nothing. Pete called 911. I had never known that before. Pete had never talked about it. It must have been so traumatic for him. But that night, those memories were a distant past. Pete was beaming, as picture after picture was taken with him and individual family members—Pete, the miracle man!

Pete's Carepage: March 1, 2007 @ 9:14 p.m.

Lots of conversation between the Cleveland Clinic, the Cincinnati doc and us throughout the last week. Praise God for this not-smallest of miracles—docs working well together! The only consensus is that the area in Pete's brain that is affected has progressed worse since the last MRI. The injured area is larger and the clinic was concerned with a new spot (but contiguous to the injured area) that appeared in this MRI that is in the "bridge" between the right and left side of the brain. A second PET scan that was done this past Monday showed a positive tumor result. However, PET scans aren't the most reliable in the brain, and the both the clinic docs and the Cincinnati doc were quick to say that this might not be a tumor at all, but a more injured area. So they both agreed on a plan. Pete's dosage level of steroids is increased. Tumors don't respond to steroids, but injured tissue does. So "smaller or the same" at the next MRI at the end of March is the desired outcome!

Bill has been doing healing touch on Pete very intensely over the last days. The archangels Uriel, Raphael and Gabriel all showed up two days in a row! So with the archangels to help Pete do battle—and all of you lifting us up in prayer—as Pete says—it's "just incredible!" How lucky we are to have such love and support around us. THANK YOU. So keep praying—pray that the cancer cell activity doesn't return and that Pete's brain will heal.

We have a "no worry" zone until the end of March. So we're off again to the sports car races—this time to the 12 Hours of Sebring in Sebring, Florida! (Find that on a map!) Pete is feeling great and there is just that small hint of spring in the air. We take hope in the coming of spring—and in the belief that God will show his glory still, just as He has been doing in Pete's recovery.

At that visit with Dr. Albright, we talked about the possible treatment of Pete's continuing necrosis through the use of a hyperbaric oxygen chamber. Hyperbaric oxygen therapy (HBOT) could be done at one of the local hospitals, or at the Air Force hospital in Wright-Patt Air Force Base in Dayton, Ohio. There are not many sites where these chambers are found, since they are expensive. The principle of HBOT was to push oxygen into Pete's brain to see if the increased dose of oxygen would have a positive effect on healing the dead brain tissue. If the amount of dead tissue was reduced, the damage this dead tissue was doing to the rest of Pete's brain would also be alleviated.

The way this treatment worked was that the HBO chamber was pressurized with pure oxygen. Normally when we breathe, we receive about twenty per cent oxygen and eighty percent nitrogen. "The increased pressure within the chamber and the increase in the oxygen level dissolved the oxygen into the blood and other tissues up to twenty times the normal concentration," Dr. Albright said.

"Necrosis has an eighty percent positive response to HBOT, based on my experience with damage from radiation treatment. But there is still the chance that it's not necrosis, and it might not be dead tissue from radiation. You would need to go to one of these centers five days a week for three months. Each treatment or dive is about two and one half hour hours long. You would need to have sixty dives for it to be effective."

Pete and I both looked at each other. "Huge time commitment," we said. Even more than the radiation treatments.

"But there are few negative side effects," Dr. Albright said. "It's primarily just your lungs and ears at risk from the increased pressure. There is an attendant with you at all times in case your body reacts to the compression and subsequent de-compression."

The clinic was not as enthusiastic about the HBOT treatment, and both doctors agreed to increase the steroid dosage initially as a way to control the inflammation and the spread of the necrosis. Pete and I weren't opposed to the HBOT, but we also hesitated to give up another three months of our lives to daily treatments. Pete had so many other things on his list he wanted to do! And I wanted him to be able to do all of it! So we suspended this treatment decision until we got back from Florida and the Sebring sports car race.

Sometimes the roller coaster of uncertainty would not be spread out over weeks and months, but could occur within a day or days. One incident I recall happened the day my father was having surgery to remove the mass found in his colon. Pete and I were in the waiting room with the family when I looked at Pete and saw that his eye was bloodshot. I looked at my sister and asked her if she had her blood pressure cuff with her. I don't know why I noticed it at that moment.

Mary Jo took Pete's blood pressure and it was high: 180/120. We called his primary care doctor, and got orders to come to his office immediately. The doctor had no idea what would have spiked Pete's blood pressure. He prescribed strong medicine, Clonidine, to bring Pete's pressure down. For the next six days, I monitored Pete's pressure every three hours during the day. It would go high and then dip way low. I had to call the doctor a number of times so he could adjust the dosage. The doctor was worried this strong medicine might take Pete's blood pressure too low. He gave me parameters: Call if Pete's BP (blood pressure) is below 100 or pulse is below 50. One day I called twice and he finally stopped the Clonidine. He moved Pete back to the same medication he had been on before all the brain surgeries had begun. Pete stabilized. No one knew the cause. Living with uncertainty.

Crossroads created a prayer experience for all its members right before Easter. It was experiential. We were given headsets and an audio CD that led us through the experience, focusing on a different topic in each room. Pete and I went through it together. In one room there were rocks, and we were encouraged to identify something in our lives that we grasped too tightly, and to give it up and throw the rock into the makeshift pond.

This was my conversation with God in that room: *Pete is the rock that I grasp too tightly. I want to hold onto that rock. I can't throw it into the pond. Why? Who could take better care of Pete than You? No One! He's yours anyway. He is your child; he belongs to you and I am just lucky enough to have a little time with him. He comes from you and he will return to you, and I need to not so desperately hold on. I release Pete to You. I trust in your love of him. You love him so! You are his healer. You protect him from evil. You will never abandon him. You will always be with him. Your presence is guaranteed. And your presence is enough. I need not carry this burden. I cannot control the outcome for Pete. I can influence you in my prayer for him. I can love him and look out for his needs as your servant. I can be your arms and legs in loving him. And what an honor. But you are teaching me to hold lightly. Give me a gentle touch.*

20

The Last Trip

We got back from our trip to Glacier and Yellowstone toward the end of July 2007. We started using light weights to build up Pete's strength, and we walked almost every day down in our favorite park by the river. I noticed that Pete's symptoms were getting worse. He was dragging his right foot more than ever when he walked. One night he couldn't remember how to make mashed potatoes, but then it all came back to him as he started to do it. Blood vessels kept breaking in Pete's eyes. His ability to process information seemed to be slowing down, although he still understood everything. His response times were just slower. His reading and writing capabilities were worse. I started watching him get a vacant stare more often. I felt like a failure as a caregiver, because Pete was getting worse. I knew intellectually that was ridiculous, but my feelings were my feelings. That performance comparison habit was a hard thing to break. The one thing that Pete did complain about was his vision. Repeated trips back to the eye doctor facilitated a slight adjustment in his prescription, which seemed to satisfy for awhile, but not really fix the problem.

I called the project manager for the IL-13 clinical trial, hoping to get some answers to Pete's worsening condition. My thought was to talk to other IL-13 patients to compare experiences.

Deb told me, "Pete is the last and the longest survivor of the IL-13 treatment without another intervention in our study. He may be the longest survivor in the country."

"Oh," I said. "Are you telling me there is no one to talk to?"

She was silent. I first felt pride in Pete's stamina. Then I felt shame. When I told Pete what Deb told me, he just looked at me with deep hurt and sadness in his eyes. He didn't say a word. I kicked myself for even sharing that information with him. Deb also told us that the pharmacy company which sponsored the IL-13 clinical trial had closed the study. The results were not significantly better than other, less-expensive treatments.

It was hard for me to have any hope. The steroids Pete was taking to control the inflammation kept making his body weaker. Other treatment options were not very attractive. On August 8, 2007, Pete gave up driving. I felt sad and relieved. Others had been pressuring me to keep Pete from driving. I refused to deny him. I trusted him. He was a very cautious man, and he would know when it wasn't safe. And he did.

The August round of MRI and doctor visits and reviews showed no change. Same injury pattern; the enhanced area was not growing. Dr. Albright wanted to do something to treat Pete! He tried to convince us. "Injury begets injury," he explained.

He drew us a circle showing how Pete's vascular system first sends a trigger; Pete's immune system tries to fight it, which leads to inflammation of the tissues. The steroids react and control the inflammation, but the vascular system is still sending the signal. Dr. Albright thought that if Pete took Avastin, the vascular trigger would be reduced or decreased.

The clinic was not enthused about the use of Avastin for Pete. They called it an off-label solution for brain cancer, and still risky. Avastin was a drug that had been approved for breast, lung and colon cancer. Dr. Albright had good experience with it for treating recurring brain tumors. He was using it off-label. Avastin worked by slowing the growth of new blood vessels, which in turn reduced the blood supply to tumors. Tumors can't grow without an aggressive blood supply.

It turned out Dr. Albright was right, just ahead of the experts. In June 2009, Avastin got approval for treating recurring glioblastoma tumors. So Dr. Albright was leading the way. As Genentech mentioned in the press release, it was "the first new treatment for glioblastoma in more than a decade."

"I don't want to do anything different right now," Pete said. "This is my decision and no one else's," Pete emphasized. "I am so happy with you. I love having you this close to me."

At the same time that Pete's symptoms were getting worse, he'd surprise me. He painted the front gate to our deck one day. It must have been 90 degrees. He sat on a little stool with a bottle of water at his side, and painted the gate carefully, brush by brush stroke. Right next to that gate, we stored wood for the fireplace. He moved all the wood on the deck to find any bugs, and check for termites. At those moments, it was hard for me to believe that Pete's tumor was back.

One night we played the DVD of the Rolling Stones concerts. He and I sat on our couch singing along with the Stones and drinking wine. He remembered all the words to the songs! During the concert, Pete jumped up from the couch and started dancing. He beckoned me to join him. I did. He was ecstatically happy.

Pete was motivated by planning and taking trips. At the end of August, we made a weekend visit to Washington, DC to see Steve and Kathy. We flew this time. I can still close my eyes and see the precious look on Pete's face as his son met him at the airport. They embraced. Pete's eyes misted over. His son, his precious treasure.

Kathy was running a marathon in Annapolis, Maryland, the weekend we visited. Kathy gave us a great excuse to go back to one of our favorite cities. Many a night Pete and I had eaten dinner at the Chart House in Annapolis. The restaurant was right on the water. In the summer, Wednesday nights sported a sailboat regatta. We talked of our memories of the colors of those spinnakers catching the setting sun. A glorious sight! And Pete remembered the garlic dip—his favorite! And I relished the she crab soup, which was the best I had ever tasted anywhere in this country. We loved the soup so much that Pete years ago had convinced the chef to give us the recipe. Which he did. We still joke with Jack and Judith about the New Year's Eve with them on a cold Cincinnati night when Judith and Pete made the Chart House crab soup for us. Pete forgot the recipe was restaurant-sized. He made three gallons of soup that night!

Pete continued to amaze me with his independence and lack of fear, even in the face of walking difficulty and word-finding challenges. One day, while I was away from the house at a meeting, Pete went out walking in our neighborhood by himself. He didn't tell me his plan beforehand. When I returned, I asked how his day was. He told me he had walked the neighborhood and visited a friend. He couldn't find the name of who he had visited. I had guessed it was his frequent lunch partner, Mike Gendron, who also lived in Mount Adams.

Pete said, "Yes."

"How was your visit?" I asked.

"I was kicked out," Pete said. "He had a bad cold so he asked me to leave after about twenty minutes."

I laughed, delighted in him. "How did you find him?" I asked.

Pete looked at me kind of stupidly and said "Well, I knew where he lived, so I just decided to stop by."

Pete had a napkin in his hand that had a drawing of a terminal in the local airport, and an arrow that showed in Mike's handwriting, "Mike's plane." Mike G. was a pilot. Mike G. told me later that Pete had asked him what it would take to fly with him. He told him "a simple request is all." So Mike G. booked a flight with Pete.

"It was one of the best flying days I have ever had in Cincinnati," Mike said.

I smiled and thought, ah yes. You were with Pete. You got the blessings he gets. Yes—the most perfect flying day you have ever had in Cincinnati and Mike has probably been flying for over twenty-five years. It's because you were with Pete!

Mike G. said, "I gave Pete the full 'magilla' from preflight weather, to complete preflight of the aircraft, to talking to air traffic control. For the twenty minutes before engine start, he smiled, listened, and seemed to enjoy every detail. As I crawled around the plane I showed

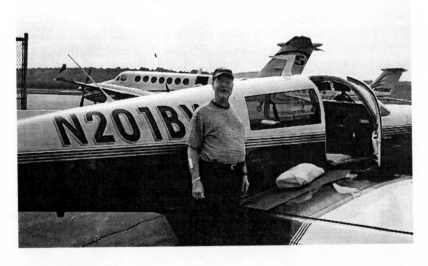

Pete and Mike G.'s plane

him the control surfaces, connections that I was checking, and fluids." Mike smiled. "Pete seemed like a race car driver appreciating each step of a safe preflight.

"Once the engine started, we donned the headphones and enjoyed the dialogue with air traffic control. During the engine run-up to full power while holding on the taxiway, Pete seemed to enjoy the noise, and the engine straining against the brakes holding us secure on the runway."

I mentioned to Pete, "If for any reason you want to return, I can do so on a moment's notice—air traffic control is very cooperative when asked to do so." Pete nodded.

"We flew over Clermont County Airport, East Fork Lake, and circled for a few minutes at about three thousand feet and one hundred and fifty miles per hour. Pete hadn't said a word up to this point, but beamed the broadest grin and happiest eyes that I'd ever seen. When I asked him if he wanted to pilot the plane, he turned with that broad grin, and only shook his head as if to say 'Why would I clutter this wonderful experience with work such as controlling the plane?' He returned to scanning the lake, patchwork fields and broad blue sky. I asked, 'Are you ready to return?' Pete quietly nodded yes as if to say 'mission accomplished.'

"I checked with air traffic control to get permission to fly up the river and over your house in Mount Adams. Once again, a broad smile and not a word spoken. We switched over to Lunken ATC and I mentioned we would be landing at about ninety miles per hour. Wheels touched down and we taxied to the hangar."

Mike G. told me, "I think Pete didn't say a word because he couldn't stop smiling long enough for words. I don't think I have ever seen a happier or more contented passenger, who could not stop gazing out the windows as the landscape passed beneath our wings. What a wonderful trip for me," Mike G. said with love in his eyes.

After the flight, Pete told Mike G "Be sure and tell Kathy how much I enjoyed the trip." He also mentioned that he had driven his cars as fast as we had flown. Can you imagine?

"But a Porsche would do that, wouldn't it?" Mike G. asked.

"Yes, a Porsche would and did, Mike," I said.

Pete was driving. He remembered.

In September, Pete and I made it to the Cincinnati Bengals football game with our nephew Caleb and his friend, Bo. The game was packed. Huge crowds and hot. I was amazed by how well Pete navigated through the crowds with these two young boys, who were walking fast and not paying any attention to their uncle's situation. Pete didn't flinch.

I was now driving Pete to and from his school board meetings and Roundtable meetings. He never hesitated about going. He'd call me on his cell phone when he was ready for pick up, which was a feat in itself—just for him to remember our phone number. I only got a call once in those months from the principal of one of the schools, saying Pete was ready to come home.

When we took our last trip we didn't know it was going to be our last one. But appropriately so, it was Pete's favorite place—Napa and Sonoma wine country in California. Mary Jo and Mike came with us, so Pete would now be able to show them Napa, just like he had introduced them to Daytona and the twenty-four-hour race. Mary Jo, Mike and I also wanted to visit Yosemite while we were out there, and Pete agreed to come along.

Pete was so excited about going to Napa again! He started planning our stay well in advance. We had been to Napa and Sonoma a number of times before, and he had carefully recorded on a pink index card all the wineries we had visited, and when we had gone. Pete had a single white piece of folio paper that had a number of columns with headings: 92, 93, 94, 95, 96, 97 and 98. Those numbers represented the Robert Parker wine rating system. Wines in the 96–100 category were extraordinary; 90–95 were outstanding wines. Pete read a number of wine magazines that used the Parker rating system. Pete would only note those wines on his sheet of paper that achieved Parker's rating of at least 90 and also met his own criteria—"could be bought for $50.00 or less." He'd record those wines in each of the columns on his folio paper, and then would use this list in planning our next trip to the wineries. He had built his list over the last seven to eight years. He would update it regularly.

Since writing had become difficult for him, Pete had resorted to tearing out the pages in his wine magazines that described the wines that met his criteria. These now needed to be put on his list. He needed to do it so we could plan our visit. He had a pretty good stack of magazine pages to sort through.

One afternoon, we updated the list. Pete tried writing the names of the wineries in the appropriate column, and his scribbling next to his nice, neat previous entries led to a scream of frustration.

"I can't do this anymore," he cried out. "Look at this writing. It is awful!"

I took over the recorder's job. "Is this the column where you want me to put this wine?" I asked, with not a lot of patience.

"No, no, no," Pete yelled in frustration.

We sat in silence. His frustration mounted. My sadness overwhelmed me. We took a break. Pete's list got updated.

Pete planned our Napa and Sonoma trip in these categories: our favorite wineries in Napa and Sonoma where we wanted to take Mary Jo and Mike; new wineries we wanted to visit; and then our favorite restaurants. As Pete and I talked, I recorded where we wanted to go. Pete was satisfied. We placed this plan right under that single sheet of white folio paper with all his ratings. Pete couldn't wait to go; neither could I.

From my prayer journal: September 3, 2007

Things are changing, Lord, with Pete. I see his decline, all the things he can't do. I observe all the new symptoms. It's all bad news right now. Pete's decline makes me sad. It makes me angry at you. Somehow I feel like you are disappointing us. How stupid is that! I know you do not cause Pete's decline. But it does make me feel like you are not rescuing him. He is getting worse. The disease may be getting worse and you are not intervening. I believe you could. But you are not in the way I want you to. I am a spoiled child. Angry and pouting. I am embarrassed.

And you tell me, "What don't you understand?" just like you told the disciples when the storm was rocking the boat. "I am here. I love Pete. I love you. I am here. Trust me. I know what is best for the both of you. Open your eyes so you can see. Trust in me and my power. Trust in my love of you both. And I'll lead you through."

And I say, "I know your ways are not our ways. Your love and presence is enough. Teach me to see Pete as you see him, not his decline, but his beauty. I know you have a special place in your heart for him. You are close to those suffering. You give him your special blessings. And you are enough."

Bill came and did Healing Touch on Pete. For the first time in a long time, Pete's right arm showed full energy. "You are like my brother," Bill said to Pete. "I am very tuned into your energy fields. All energy is intelligent. Your energy fields actually give me direction. You are pure and holy and a powerful energy."

As I walked Bill out to the car, he said to me, "I have learned a lot from Pete."

"Yes, I have to," I said.

"I always feel a sense of calm and peace when I work on Pete. I'm not sure I could be that calm, given what Pete has been through."

"You are such a good source of encouragement for Pete and for me," I told Bill.

Bill laughed. "Who is encouraging who?" he said. "Pete told me today, 'I am grateful to be alive every day.' How amazing is that! He is always calm. Positive. Peaceful. Appreciative. He always says thank you. How special Pete is!" Bill said almost in a chuckle.

I hugged Bill. "Thank you," I said.

I watched Bill pull away from the curb. I thought about what Pete had said to me the night before at dinner, "I might not get my directions, but I have a wonderful woman!" I smiled and thought, *and I have a wonderful man. And this is God's presence in Pete—what I see—what Bill sees—what is between us. This is what it means,* I thought, *to see God's glory shining all around.*

Pete's Carepage: September 13, 2007 @ 10:15 PM EDT

More prayers, please... Pete's latest scans were definitely worse than last month's. The injured area has grown, spreading down toward the back of Pete's brain and crossing over to the right side of his brain, which up to this point has been unaffected. Both the Cincinnati doctor and the Cleveland Clinic think it is unlikely that this "growth" is a tumor. That's the good news. But the injury is spreading and causing more damage. Obviously, the steroids are not controlling the injured area as they have been. So—time for something new. Pete has continued to be his amazing self through this. Very calm and peaceful. Still focused on every new day and appreciating the opportunity each day brings.

The good news is there is consensus among the doctors to try Avastin to treat the injured area. (Another small miracle, given their disagreement on this less than six weeks ago.) Avastin is a man-made antibody that stops blood flow to the injured area. Avastin is used predominantly for colon cancer, but our Cincinnati doc has been "experimenting" successfully with a few patients to use Avastin for damaged brain tissue. Clearly this treatment is experimental, but the truth, I have come to realize, is that the doctors really don't have any more proven treatments to try. Pete is a "one-of-a-kind"—which we always knew! (Smile.) So we need to try something, and even though there are risks, Pete is willing to take them. Avastin will also let Pete get off the steroids eventually, which will be a good thing.

One thing Pete was absolutely clear about was that he wasn't going to start ANY treatment till we got back from our next trip. As he said, "I've got my priorities!" So tomorrow we leave for a wonderful trip to San Francisco/Napa/Yosemite. For those of you who know Pete well, you know how much he loves wine and how he has educated himself over the years about wine. He "introduced" Mary Jo and Mike to good wine, and so their request of Pete was to "show them Napa." It took Pete all of one second to say "Yes" and get excited—so off we go! As an added bonus, we get to see some of my US Bank friends in this market. So the next update will include some wine stories. Pete will start this new treatment, when we return the week of Sept. 24.

So pray for this injured area in Pete's brain to stop spreading, and if feeling "bold," ask for it to be reduced! Pray that the cancer not

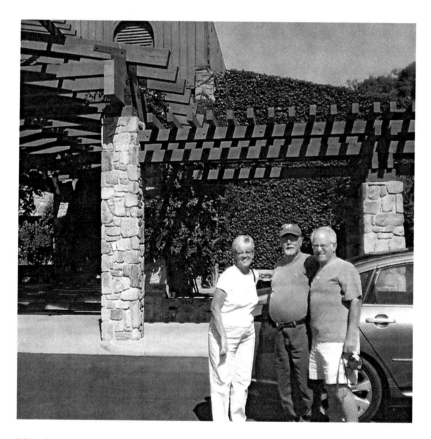

Mary Jo, Pete, and Mike in Napa

return. Pray for wisdom in our doctors. Pray that this new treatment will work, and Pete will not be harmed. Pray that Pete and I never underestimate or under-appreciate the power of our God. Your prayers and belief have made Pete strong in his battle over the last twenty months. We are humbled in knowing how much you love and support us. Thank you.

The news we got at this doctor's visit was that the injured area had gotten larger, spread toward the back of Pete's brain, and crossed over to the right side of his brain. Dr. Albright wanted to start Avastin right away. Pete wanted to wait until after the Napa trip.

"Are you afraid based on the news we got yesterday?" I asked Pete.

"No." He shook his head. "We have been here before and then things change."

"Whatever is happening in your brain is causing damage, Pete, and that damage can't be fixed. I am not sure we can wait till after the Napa trip," I said.

"But our friends want to go," Pete said.

"Mary Jo and Mike wouldn't want you to make that decision based on them," I retorted.

"What?" Pete said. "Are you against going to Napa?" he asked with some alarm, and this look of being abandoned.

"I'll do whatever you want. I trust your decision. Just don't make it based on disappointing them," I said.

A phone call from one of the people that used to work for me in San Francisco interrupted our conversation. "That was Ole calling, Pete. He says we have nine people coming to lunch with us when we arrive in San Francisco."

Pete got misty-eyed. "They are coming for you!" he said. "It's been almost two years since they worked for you and they are coming for you!"

"And to see you!" I said. "They have been following your journey on the Carepages."

"No," he said, "they are coming to see you. You'll go back and work with them again. That would be good."

I stopped arguing. I knew Pete was touched. He was proud of me, that so many people in the middle of a Friday workday would make the trip into the city to have lunch with us. I was amazed at him. We had just gotten bad news about the progression of his disease that was wreaking havoc in his brain, and he was excited because of the support I was getting. Oh my.

Pete's Carepage: October 3, 2007 @ 11:44 AM EDT

Thanks to all who prayed us safely to and back from San Francisco/Napa/Yosemite. GREAT time was had by all. Pete just loved being back in Napa. We visited ten wineries—five of our favorites to share with Mike and Mary Jo, and five new ones Pete had researched through his wine magazines. We did a sunrise hot-air balloon ride. WOW. And enjoyed lunch at two favorite spots— Auberge du Soleil and Meadowood. The weather was September's best in Napa.

Pete had three falls while we were on the trip. He can't control them and doesn't get any warning. His right side just gives way. Needless to say he is unnerved by them, and luckily, other than a few scrapes, has escaped more serious injury. Pete needs more assistance now in walking than before, and is having difficulty climbing steps and doing normal things like showering and dressing. He has lots of fight, though. Resists help—and pushes himself to do as much as he can. And is amazing as ever—never complaining—thankful for each day!

When we returned, we had another MRI which showed a slight worsening since the scan three weeks ago, but not significantly so. Pete started a new treatment on Sept. 27 which is highly experimental, called Avastin, that he will take every two weeks. He also got a port-a-cath placed in his shoulder so future treatments don't have to go through his veins. We will know the benefit of the new treatment in the next scan on October 18. The only side effect is fatigue. And Pete has been experiencing his share of that. The fatigue makes everything worse: walking, speaking, etc. He told me this morning, "It seems to be getting worse. Blah!"

Pray that this new treatment has positive benefits for Pete. Ask for protection for him so that he doesn't hurt himself, especially when falling. And as ever, I thank you for your belief in us and love and prayers for us.

P.S. Here's a good story. Pete received a prayer shawl this week from a US Banker who we hadn't heard from in twenty months. She has done five other shawls, and even though she had not sent cards or notes to us over the last twenty months, she had been praying for Pete and me faithfully, and listed us in her "prayer box." She believes in the power of prayer—and so in starting her sixth shawl she was "led" to make it for Pete. Ah—God sends angels at just the right time.

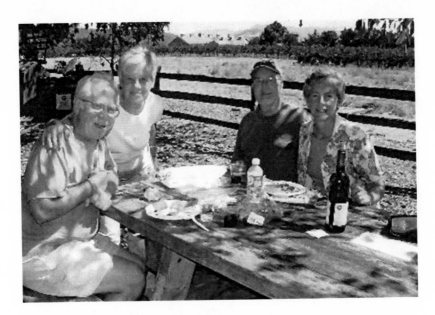

Mike, Mary Jo, Pete, and Kathy in Napa

For those of you who have been to Napa, you will recognize this picture as the picnic tables at a popular lunch spot in Napa, V. Sattui's winery. Pete surprised me the day we stopped there for our wine and cheese and fruit lunch. It was September 17, 2007. As we sat down to eat our feast, Pete pulled out of his pocket a little blue Tiffany's box and set it on the picnic table. He didn't say a word, just looked at me with such love in his eyes that I felt my heart soar. I burst into tears and crawled into his arms. It was the day before my birthday. I opened the box. A beautiful set of silver mesh earrings with a single pearl dangling from each wire was in the box. The matching necklace, I received the following day. I was so surprised, my mouth just gaped open. I kept looking at him.

"You remembered. You remembered." I kept saying. "They are beautiful. Oh Pete." And more tears.

Pete just grinned with kind of a bad boy grin, so satisfied with himself that he had pulled this off.

"How did you do this?" I asked.

Pete sat up real straight and Mike began to tell the story.

"Remember the day Pete and I went to lunch?" Mike asked me. "Well, Pete told me he wanted to go downtown to do some shopping. He couldn't tell me where he wanted to go, but I knew he knew. He directed me where to park. Then he made a beeline to the Tiffany's store. You should have seen him with the salesperson," Mike said, laughing. Pete just smiled his bad-boy grin.

"Well, this salesperson started stalking Pete. Pete was walking like he was on a mission, hovering over the jewelry cases and peering into them. She kept saying, 'Do you like this one?' or 'What about this one?' or 'This is pretty!'

"Pete shook his head as in 'no' and kept walking. Finally, he stopped. He didn't say a word. He pointed to these earrings in the case, and the salesperson brought them out. Pete smiled. He had found the perfect gift. This time Pete shook his head as in 'yes' as the salesperson asked, 'Do you like these?' Pete reached for his wallet and took out his credit card and paid for the set. Then he looked at me with a real satisfied look and said 'lunch!'"

I looked at Pete and asked, "So how did you get these to Napa without me finding them?" I had packed our suitcases with Pete's assistance, and never uncovered the blue boxes. Pete just smiled and looked at Mike. I knew there was a secret there, and neither of them was talking.

Pete's falls during this trip scared all of us. The first fall was the first night we arrived. We went up to the bar at the Top of the Mark in San Francisco. Pete seemed to have stumbled where the carpet joined the tile at the entrance. He didn't fall all the way; Mike caught him. We brushed it off. I had been charging ahead of Pete, and I got mad at myself, making note to always walk on his right side. Always meant always.

A few days later, we were at the Auberge du Soleil restaurant for lunch. It was a small place and crowded. Pete lost his balance and careened toward the tables. Mary Jo and I were right there, and we caught him as he fell into an empty table. Other than a small disruption to the guests and Pete's embarrassment, no harm was done.

The third fall happened toward the end of our Napa trip. We had just finished breakfast and left the hotel room. All four of us were walking on the sidewalk heading toward the car, and Pete fell down fast, headfirst. His glasses flew off. He didn't catch himself at all, landing squarely on his face. Blood spurt out on his brand new t-shirt and Mike's, who had rushed to Pete's assistance. Mike had bought Pete and himself matching t-shirts from the Plumpjack winery we had visited the day before. It was Pete's favorite winery.

"What happened, Pete?" Mary Jo asked with concern.

Pete couldn't find the words. "My side just gave out," Pete stammered.

"You had no warning?" Mary Jo quizzed.

Pete shook his head. Mary Jo and I had been on each side of him, and were frustrated because it happened so fast, we couldn't react. Mary Jo checked for broken bones, and Pete looked fine other than the scrapes on his arms and face. Most normal people would call it a day at that point and take a rest. Not Pete. He shrugged it off. We cleaned him up right there on the sidewalk, because it was too much effort for him to walk back into the hotel room. Pete was relieved that his glasses hadn't broken. I cleaned them, and he put them back on. He was ready to go. "We have wineries to visit!" he exclaimed. "Let's go."

Mary Jo and Mike left for home a day before we did. Ole had invited Pete and me to his wedding in Carmel. I told Pete we didn't have to stay, and could go home with Mary Jo and Mike. It had already been a long trip. He wouldn't hear of leaving. He stayed for me.

We drove to Carmel the morning of the wedding. I stopped at a gas station in Gilbert, California, to get a bottle of water. When I got back in the car, Pete said he needed to go to the bathroom, and fast! I asked the attendant where the bathrooms were, and he pointed to a Port-A-Pot in the parking lot. Pete couldn't wait to find a better restroom. This would have to do. As we climbed into the Port-A-Pot and were pulling his pants down, he couldn't hold it any longer and a runny stool cascaded all over the pot, Pete's underwear and Pete. Pete was in dress slacks and a suit coat. I was in a dress and hose and heels. There was no running water. The sun coming through the Port-A-Pot gave us both a garish turquoise hue.

I bolted out the door, and saw a customer waiting to use the pot. I rushed by him, desperate to buy some wet-and-dries. I sighed in relief. The store carried them. Two packages later, I returned. I can't imagine how Pete had to be feeling. Vulnerable. Embarrassed. Just sitting there in a mess waiting for me.

I opened the Port-A-Pot door and kissed him on the top of his head. We looked at each other and realized the craziness of the situation. We burst into laughter. That Pot was a-rockin'! The customer outside finally gave up waiting. It took us a good twenty minutes to clean up, and we proceeded to the wedding just short a pair of underwear. Pete had to be exhausted. He didn't flinch or want to turn back. We made it to the wedding, which was held at the historic, beautiful Le Playa

Hotel in Carmel by the Sea. The hotel sat on a hill. The ceremony was in the gardens. There were no banisters, and the sidewalk was uneven brick. Pete climbed those steps, slowly, one by one. He was his gracious self, smiling and chatting to those we knew.

After the wedding, we made it back to our hotel without incident. We cleaned up, and I was surprised when Pete said he wanted to go down to the hotel lobby to watch football and eat some dinner. I couldn't believe he still had energy. It was such a normal thing for us to do. I treasured that evening.

When we got back to Cincinnati, it was Pete's birthday. Paula had organized a family party, and everyone was there. My nephews came in from Atlanta and Louisville. At Paula's request, each person had given her little sayings or items that represented Pete to them. Paula had organized all their comments into a collage with pictures of Pete, his favorite sayings and the things he loved. Paula framed it and had each person sign the back.

Pete was so touched. His eyes misted as he read the words. Leaky tears ran down his cheeks. That collage was so him: CEO of the Angus Group, Captain of My Destination, Father, Husband, Napa and Plumpjack and grilling and salmon and garlic and ice cream sundaes. The Rolling Stones and Porsches and the 24 Hours of Daytona and Le Mans. Snipes of Pete's favorite sayings: "So Far, So Good," "Hey, Hey, Hey," and "I appreciate every day!" made it perfect. Pete would not let that collage leave his sight. He propped it up so he could see it from his favorite chair. It stayed there close to him for the rest of his life.

I wrote him this letter for his sixty-second birthday. It appears here just as I gave it to him in large type so he could read it. I read the letter to him at breakfast. I read it to him in between my leaky tears.

To Pete on your 62nd birthday.

I love you Pete Nadherny for all the qualities that are YOU.

I respect your fight and determination. Your fight to live each day all the way. How full of thanks you are! I am humbled.

I respect how you never focus on your health problems or your challenges. I ask you how you are feeling and with defiance, you say "fine" and immediately turn and

ask me "how are YOU feeling?!" just like there is no difference in the magnitude of those 2 questions.

I love your courage. "I have fun everyday," you say." I
don't know how many days I have left so I have fun each
day no matter what."

I love to watch you think. The look on your face when
you are calculating a tip at the restaurant or signing a
check or writing a note on a card to one of our sons. The
pain-staking care. The concentration you give the task.

I love the way you laugh. Laughing as we pull into
your favorite winery-Plumpjack—and laughing with
delight when you decide to buy and ship one home. I
love the way Mike W makes you laugh—at anything and
everything. Doesn't matter. You laugh a lot. And I love
you for it. And you have taught me how to laugh.

I love the way your eyes get 'misty' when you are
touched by someone else's kindness to you. Like Steve &
Kathy's walk with you around their neighborhood and
later you said, "They did that for me. They did that for
me."

And I love the way you love me so much that your eyes
mist-up when others show kindness to me! After 2 years,
you said, "all those people getting together for lunch to
see you!"

I love the way you are always the "gentleman." You can
barely walk but I must proceed you and you must open
the door for Mary Jo. You say "thank you" for every
courtesy extended you by anyone—hospital staff/wait-
resses/airline stewards/family/friends. You have thanked
me a million times in 2 years. And I have heard you
thank others a million times, too.

I love the anger in your eyes when you have been
wronged. Pure, intense, clear and blue steel. "You always
do this," you said loudly (not quite a scream). "Let me
finish the story please!"

I love the way you love me and the look in your eyes
when you surprised me the day before my birthday with
the blue box on the picnic table at VSattui's in Napa.

I love the way you look out for me—all the time. Crossing the street at the airport or forgetting my purse at the restaurant or pointing at a shoelace untied.

Most of all I respect your graciousness in being cared for by others. For a proud, successful and independent man to accept so gracefully the help of others has to be at times excruciating. And it is your humility and appreciation that makes me marvel and feel so lucky to have this chance to partner with you.

Pete Nadherny—YOU have saved my life on more than one occasion. How much more meaning could you ever wring from life than to know you have done the most noble act-giving your life for another's. And not just my life but you have saved many others lives all along the way.

I love you because you are the best husband any "girl" could ever have and the best partner to journey with through life.

You are a most honorable man. I admire and respect you and love you with all my heart. Happy 62nd year.

From my prayer journal: September 26, 2007

How graced we are to celebrate Pete's birthday today! He is 62. I wasn't sure we would see this day together. Thank you, Lord. Sing praise to you! Bless Pete especially today with your presence. Deepen his understanding of how much you love him, and deepen his faith and trust in you. Protect him from the evil one and all bad spirits. Grace our day together. May your presence be here.

21

Doing the Dance

Pete and Mike got inspired after our trip to Napa to make their own wine. Pete had gone to a winemaking class years before, and had made a couple of cases of chardonnay. He had always intended to make a second batch of his favorite red wine the next time. So Mike found a place where he and Pete could make red wine. Pete was so excited. They started as soon as we got back from Napa. The grapes were imported. Pete and Mike tested each of them and then chose two varietals. They made a big batch which would give each of us about sixty bottles. After the batch was made, the fermentation process began. Pete would take me out to the winemaking place to check on his batch periodically. Since I had never been there, Pete directed me and I drove. The winemaker was always so kind to us. Pete showed me his batches in big white plastic containers, and I felt like I was being shown a valuable piece of art in process.

Pete and Mike decided to call their wine "Riverview Estates" after their homes, which both overlooked the river. Their label sported pictures we had taken in the Tetons. We had such fun the night we bottled it! Mike, Mary Jo, Pete and I brought a picnic lunch, and although the setting was not as nice as Napa, we had a grand time. Mike siphoned the wine into the bottles, Mary Jo and I did the cork-

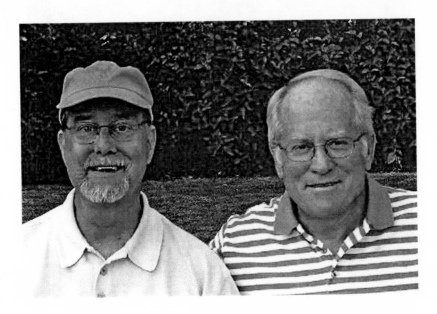

Pete and Mike

ing, Pete did the sealing, all while drinking our wine and nibbling. Thanks to our vintners, Pete and Mike, we now had our own taste of Napa forever in our homes in Ohio.

Things were getting worse for Pete. He was losing his balance more frequently. He fell a few more times at home, once cracking his head on the granite countertop in our dressing area. We'd sit on the floor together after these falls, and just look at each other before we began the challenging process of getting him up.

"What are you thinking," I asked Pete after one of these falls.

"I am just mad," he said.

Bleeding came with the falls, but no broken bones. A continual blessing. Answered prayers to protect Pete!

Through the month of October, things kept getting worse. Pete couldn't sign his name anymore when the bank sent documents over to our home. I signed for him and then initialed it. Some days he was so exhausted he wouldn't shower or shave. He started bleeding from his rectum. Pete had started Avastin as soon as we got home from California. Avastin can create bleeding in lots of places. Pete's nose bled. His arms bled from any little bump.

Pete turned down an invitation from Craig to go out on the boat in late October, because he didn't have confidence in his balance. Pete never before had turned down a boating invitation! He told me about the conversation with Craig.

"Our tomatoes last night were mad," Pete said.

"They were bad?" I asked.

"No, mad," Pete said again. "Our boater. When he called and I told him we weren't going, he said bye and hung up."

"Do you mean Craig? He called yesterday?" I asked.

"Yes. And he was mad. Said okay and hung up after I told him we weren't going."

Pete was distraught that he had disappointed Craig. I assured him that Craig understood.

"You know Craig, Pete; he was just being his normal, matter-of-fact, practical self."

Pete just stared at me with a pained look. I started not being able to understand everything Pete said to me. This was the first time I had this experience since right after his surgery. It scared me. I could tell he understood everything said to him, but I couldn't always decipher his message back. We tried to make the guessing of words fun. Like a game of charades. Pete was funny. He'd laugh at himself. He'd chase my fear away with his humor. As he struggled for words, he used expressions we called, "Peteisms."

Pete's favorite Cincinnati Reds baseball player at the time was Xavier Valentine, the Reds catcher. When he came up to bat while we were watching a Reds ballgame, Pete would say, "Here's the fireman."

We went to visit a new and architecturally avant-garde building with my mom at a United Way reception. Pete exclaimed the next morning: "Quite frankly, that building we were in last night wasn't that much. And where it was! But one thing about grandma (my mother), she fits in anywhere whether she likes it or not."

"Do you think the church will add another lap?" Pete asked one morning when we passed a construction site. "All I remember is talking about the electric bill," Pete said on our visit to check his wine. "I have my priorities right!"

We were having a new roof put on our house and Pete told me one morning when the workers were hanging the gutter on the back of our house, "I hope they get the carpet down today."

It was lightning one night while we were sitting on our deck. "I will go in and just say I want two umbrellas," Pete said.

"Bring me the coffee bill so in case anyone rings, I'll have it here." This meant that Pete wanted the phone next to him.

"You are not giving anyone a small lawyer" he scolded me, which I think meant, don't give any money away.

"My eyes are frosted," Pete said, taking his hand and drawing a circle around his eyes and forehead.

"Are they leaking?" I asked.

"No," Pete said, "heated."

"Throw out the ink," Pete would exclaim as he got rid of stuff he had been saving. One day we threw out almost seventy-five baseball caps. He was quite satisfied with himself!

"This is the last day to give witness," Pete said with tears in his eyes. That comment was made the day we found out his tumor was back.

In the morning, I would wash Pete's face as soon as he woke up. I'd get the washcloth nice and warm, and bring it to him while he was still in bed. It was one of our morning routines. He'd smile with a contented look and say "Ah, this is the best." One morning, instead of saying that, he surprised himself and said "making love," and his eyes sparked up. And I smiled with him.

We would pray at every meal. Sometimes I would lead the prayer, and sometimes Pete would. I remember at breakfast one morning: "Lord, thanks," Pete said. "Everything has changed and I so appreciate what it has put on you."

As it got harder and harder to express himself, Pete talked less and less. But Pete fought to keep going. He attended every school board and CEO Roundtable meeting. He went to a big public fundraising event I was in charge of, and walked in on his own, albeit slowly. He greeted people and shook hands a lot.

At home, he always joined me in the kitchen to help prepare dinner. He snapped green beans, cleaned the corn on the cob, and cut up lettuce. He joined me in cleaning up, drying the dishes and putting them away. He always squeezed my orange juice every morning, even if he had to stretch up over the counter from his wheelchair to do it. And amazing as he was, he found a way to carry the morning paper to the breakfast table while he used his walker.

I went out one day to do grocery shopping, and when I returned home I found Pete sitting on the portable toilet with the lid down. He was a mess. "I am sorry, I am sorry," he kept saying.

"It's not your fault, Pete. It's not your fault," I said as I held him and we both cried. He had tried to make it to the toilet, but he didn't have the strength to get himself on it properly. I decided from that day forward I would never leave him alone, even if only for a few hours.

And that's when our life changed again. We were dancing now. I literally gave up doing anything else other than being with and caring for Pete. No more household tasks. No more running out. Pete led the dance and I followed. Step over step, hour by hour, day by day. Although others saw him as painstakingly slow and clumsy in his movements, we were graceful and light on our feet. We could hear the music playing! And we danced and danced from morning to night. It was okay to be finishing morning showers at noon. It was okay to sit for an hour after dinner and do nothing. It was okay to crawl into each other's arms to nap on the couch. Once in a while, my multitasking self stumbled. But only for a moment. I got back in step and the dance continued.

I started asking others for more help. And help poured in. Nora and Tom brought us firewood; Christine bought our groceries; Paula helped me clean. Lots of visitors: boat-friend Craig and Barbara; Missy from Crossroads, the Snows. I wanted our home to be a joyful and pleasant place. I wanted laughter to ring all the time, and smiles to be present.

I had been looking at things wrong. I had been constantly evaluating whether Pete was going backward or forward. I was valuing our life and my care giving based on that answer. But it was the wrong question. Instead of "Is Pete doing better today?" the question was: "Are we being the best we can be today? Are we letting his glory shine?" Our dance was about taking each day, and embracing it as it unfolded. Pete led me to the right rhythm. I just had to get in step with him. And I did. And we danced and danced and danced. Every day unfolded like a flower, and I was learning not to crush the bloom.

On October 18, 2007, we visited Dr. Albright again to review Pete's MRI results. As we looked at the scan together, the bad white stuff in Pete's brain had not gotten any smaller. The Avastin had not had any effect. Dr. Albright concluded that it must be tumor cells keeping the Avastin from having any positive change. He concluded that the tumor was back. War was on. Dr. Albright roared like a lion! Aggressive chemotherapy was now in order. Temodar, an oral chemotherapy, was to begin immediately, and Pete's first dose of CPT-11, a strong chemotherapy administered intravenously, would begin Monday. The Cleveland Clinic called and confirmed Dr. Albright's assessment. The tumor was back.

From my prayer journal: October 23, 2007

What can I say to you now? It seems as if you are not going to intervene in Pete's illness. You said "My silence is my invitation to you for intimacy."

I accept your sovereignty. But I still cry out like the blind man called out to you: "Jesus, Son of David, have mercy on us!" You are the healer. Give Pete your healing touch.

You reminded me this morning of how you have stayed with us through this whole journey. You stayed with us through Pete's previous suffering when he had pneumonia. You led him out of his suffering and gave us wonderful days. Such fun for us. Such a gift from you. You will lead Pete and me again.

"Don't fret" you say. "Don't you remember? I said; "Don't let your hearts be troubled or afraid. I am with you. I am with Pete. I love him more than even you love him. Trust in my love of Pete."

Give him your healing presence, Lord. Your peace and your comfort. Keep your angels with him. Help him battle this cancer. Kill the bad cancer cells. Protect his good cells. Give him his speech back. Help him express his desires.

"How long to sing this song? How long to sing this song?"

You are Pete's deliverer. Do not delay. Don't let his enemies destroy him.

22

The Tumor is Back

Welcome to a new phase of our journey. We thank all of you and each of you who have gotten us this far through your prayers and belief. We hope you will not lose heart. Stay with us now.

Both our doctor in Cincinnati and the doctors at the Cleveland Clinic agree that the most recent MRI on Pete shows a recurrence of the brain tumor. The cancer cells are back. The new treatment Pete has received over the last month, Avastin, did nothing to heal the injured areas in Pete's brain. The docs think the presence of tumor cells offset any value Pete might have received from the Avastin. So a new phase of this journey of ours will begin on Monday, Oct. 22. Pete will begin a very aggressive chemo therapy that uses Avastin with two chemo agents—CPT-11 and Temodar. The goal is to kill the cancerous tumor cells and keep this tumor from growing.

We were very disappointed with this news. But as ever, Pete's peacefulness and calm were present. He did not hesitate in making the decision to start the new treatment. "Of course, we will do this," he said. A new fight is on. Our healer, Bill, has already called on the archangels and their helpers to come help Pete with this battle. We need the warriors now! Faithfully, Bill will stay close by Pete's side to try to offset through healing touch all the negative effects of the che-motherapy.

Pete has continued to experience pretty severe weakness on his right side. He has started using a walker, and most recently a wheel-chair for any kind of distance. He has learned how to eat left-handed! Ambidextrous that guy is! But other than that he looks healthy as can be—so he is starting this new treatment with lots of strength!

At our church Crossroads service this week, we were focused on the winter season of our life—when things seem dead and we wait with hope for the spring. It is a time of waiting and stillness. "How long Lord, to sing this song" in David's words of Ps. 40.

Pray now that the chemo agents will kill these cancer cells and that the tumor will not grow. Join Bill in asking for all those warriors to help Pete win this fight! Pray for Pete's strength to withstand the neg-ative effects of the chemotherapy, and only get the positive benefit. Obviously, God has been with Pete through each of the steps of this journey, and his gifts have been abundant! We know that your prayer has showered us with this abundance, and we thank you for your faithfulness and count on your continued belief.

The first day of Pete's IV chemotherapy, Mary Jo accompanied us to the hospital. Bill and Nan came to do healing touch on Pete. Bill stopped at the door of Pete's treatment room and said "Oh," as his arms reached out to touch the air, "the angels are here!" Pete was not afraid. I was. His body was so sensitive to anything foreign; I feared the impact the chemo would have on him.

After we left the hospital after that first treatment, I asked Pete what he wanted for lunch. "Silver poor boys," he said.

"Okay," I said, thinking madly and without a clue, what is a silver poor boy? "Have we had these silver poor boys recently?" I asked.

"Yes," Pete answered.

"Did we take anyone with us when we had them?" I replied.

"No," he said.

"Are they in Hyde Park?" I asked.

"No," Pete said.

"Downtown?"

"Not exactly," Pete replied.

"Are they a sandwich?"

"Yes," and as we drove out of the hospital, Pete anxiously pointed me to turn the opposite direction from our normal route.

I complied. And then I remembered! Pete's favorite sandwich was a Greek gyro sold by a little joint called Chicago Pizza, in the neighborhood of the hospital. The gyro was wrapped in bright silver paper. "You want a gyro!" I exclaimed with delight.

Pete smiled. We stopped. He waited in the car while I ran in for the sandwiches. He gobbled his down once we got home, and then had a nap.

Pete's diarrhea continued to be bad. I was amazed that Pete showed no signs of depression or anger as things got worse and worse for him. His peace and calmness to me were signs of God's presence with him. I felt a need to call in a nurse's aide to help me, someone trained to stay with Pete if I had to leave. Pete was adamant against it. "Not yet," he said, "not yet." I backed off.

On November 4, 2007, the Crossroads community came together again to pray for Pete and me. I was a little worried before the service that no one would show up. It had been such a long road for others to follow. I was wrong to worry. Friends, our life group, our business associates, Crossroads community members, family members, our boat friend, even Pete's physical therapist, Eric, was there. I was moved to tears in gratitude. I thanked all those present, and those not there, who have prayed and ministered to us so faithfully over these last two years. Pete was touched. He was teary. I was teary.

We asked God to heal Pete. Restore Pete. We prayed together—all these followers of Christ who had hope in the Lord's power. We asked God to hear the prayers of His people. Glorify Himself in Pete's healing. "Deliver Pete and do not delay," was our prayer.

Mary Jo and Mike were our angels again. They helped us with household tasks. They swept the decks and the sidewalks. They fixed the door leading into the garage. They fixed our mail slot. To offset Pete's difficulty in climbing the stairs, Mike made an additional banister for the other side of our stairs. Now Pete had a banister on each side to brace his weak right side when going up or down. We had three sets of stairs. Mike cut and stained the wood for each set and hung them with such care. They looked perfect! Pete was so touched. Mike did such a professional job. One wouldn't even know they weren't part of the original house design. Within weeks of getting the banisters installed, Pete started having trouble climbing into our platform bed downstairs in the master bedroom. So Mike made stairs for Pete to help him get in and out of bed. They worked like a charm.

Pete's MRI results in mid-November looked slightly better from Dr. Albright's perspective. He told us that the enhancement in Pete's brain was the largest damaged area he had ever seen in his career. "But Pete has a fighting chance," he said. "Things have not gotten worse."

Pete's Carepage: November 16, 2007 @ 4:00 PM EST

For all of you who have been "storming the heavens" on our behalf, we give thanks. Keep it up. Your relentless efforts—just like that widow Jesus talked about—are bringing Pete a little relief.

Went to the Cincinnati doc yesterday and he saw an improvement in the diseased areas in Pete's brain on the MRI. Not a HUGE or dramatic improvement, but an improvement nonetheless. Two or three areas that are diseased are less dense than they were, and better yet, there's no sign of more disease growth. So he thinks the chemo is working. YEAH! He also told us that this disease is larger in size than anything he has ever seen before in his career. We are in for a "slugfest," he said. The next six months will be a battle like we have never seen. So much will depend on Pete's body "holding up" to the onslaught of the chemo over this long of a time. So far Pete has been tolerating the chemo pretty well. He is more tired than he has been, of course, and has had bouts of diarrhea. He really isn't any better since the last MRI, but he is not worse either. He is very calm. Peaceful and so positive. He laughs at me and himself a lot. And never complains. Still thankful everyday that we wake up—together!

Nutrition and continued exercise/activity are the best things we can do to help offset the chemo's effects. We also have Bill, our healer, working with Pete faithfully through all this. His healing touch really helps to ease the negative effects in the rest of Pete's body from the chemo. Bill actually comes to the hospital while Pete is getting his treatment, and works on him while his IV is going in. Pete's energy fields have been holding strong, making his body able to heal itself and recover more easily.

So—we have a fighting chance! Pete was so encouraged yesterday. He was smiling. We praised God for his continuing hand upon us. We also know we are up against a big and ugly thing. I immediately thought, as I got the news from the doc yesterday, about how many of you had prayed and are still praying for us, and your "force" is helping Pete. Your "force" is strengthening me. I am so humbled in your presence. I can see all of you lifting us up, up, up.

So pray for the chemo to continue to have positive effects on the diseased areas of Pete's brain. Pray that the cancer cells are killed

*and can't grow. Pray for Pete's endurance and his strength to with-
stand this aggressive treatment.*

*And know that we appreciate and give thanks for you every day.
Your love and support and prayer sustain us.*

The clinic was not as optimistic as Dr. Albright, seeing improvement in some areas, but a worsening in others. I had asked Pete if he
was worried about getting the MRI results, and he told me "I don't
worry about that kind of stuff anymore. If it is bad, it is bad." The
clinic thought we were crazy to be doing a steroid taper when Pete
had a scan as bad as his was. So the steroid debate continued.

Pete continued to be frustrated with his vision. He made me take
him a number of times to Lenscrafters to try to convince them to
change his prescription. "Just make it a little bit stronger," he begged.
Pete was desperate. My heart broke for Pete each time we went. His
hopes would be dashed each visit. Finally he agreed to another
appointment with his eye doctor. We went.

The eye doctor examined Pete and then said to me, not to Pete,
which made me angry, "Pete has cataracts. He would need surgery.
There was nothing he could do to change his prescription to make an
improvement." Pete was silent all the way home from the eye doctor.
He was so disappointed. Pete was not pushing ahead for cataract surgery, even though the doctor said he could safely do it even with Pete
in chemotherapy. Cataracts were another side effect of those steroids.

We went to the brain tumor support group in November, and Pete
was clearly the person in the group who was having the most difficulty. It didn't bother me at all. It was the truth of the situation, and I
didn't feel like a failure because of Pete's condition. That change in
my attitude was progress for me! Pete never struggled with this. He
went to the group in a wheelchair. He was just grateful to go. The
leader of the group commented that "we" were quite a team. We
always talked in "we," not "I," and did everything together." He was a
source of encouragement to us.

Pete pushed forward with an outside the house activity most days,
amazing as that was. I noticed the quality of his engagement in the
activity was less, though. We went to our life group at Crossroads and
Pete was silent. I wondered if he got any value out of going, but he
clearly wouldn't go if he didn't want to. He wouldn't do this for me.
We were discussing death and Mary, a member of our group, asked
Pete if he was afraid to die.

"No, I'm not," he said.

"Do you believe in Jesus?" she asked.

"Yes. I do," Pete said. That was all he said.

We kept doing our walks in the park below our house, but instead of walking a mile, Pete would make it just to the first rim of the circle in the pavement from the car. It was about eight hundred yards, and it was agonizing for him. It took such effort. I stayed close to his side.

Pete and I went to our friend Betty's sixtieth birthday party in his wheelchair. He was quiet, and I was thankful for one of our friends, Steve, who took special care for Pete that night. Pete complained to me later that when he was in a wheelchair, he was invisible to many. People talked over him. Steve paid special attention to Pete, which was a blessing.

We went to a dinner at one of our banker friend's houses to watch the Bengals game, and I noticed how most people talked around Pete now, few talked to him. He was quiet. But he did enjoy watching the game, and being with friends. He protested loudly when someone threatened to change the channel.

Thanksgiving came and my sister, Beth, hosted the family. Pete and I made pies with Mary Jo's help. Pie-baking the night before Thanksgiving was a Pete and my tradition of many years. Pete's real pleasure, though, was cooking our own turkey a couple of days later. Pete was so happy. He loved cooking turkeys, and had done so for many, many years. He managed to prepare the turkey and baste it regularly, doing it all from his wheelchair. He even carved it himself, with a little help from my right hand. By now, we were using the wheelchair in the house all the time. Pete's right leg and foot had pretty much stopped working.

We got our Christmas tree shortly after Thanksgiving from the same lot we always visited. They would deliver it to our house. Pete went with me in the car, but could not get out. I went hunting and when I found three trees that I thought Pete would like, the Christmas tree man was kind enough to haul them up to the window of the car so Pete could choose. It was the most beautiful tree I think we ever had. Stood almost twelve feet tall and was very full. We put up the Christmas lights and ornaments, with Pete sitting in a chair right next to the tree, pulling out each ornament or light strand, and handing me each one so carefully. We filled that tree with lights and hung every one of our ornaments. Normally, we always had ornaments left over. But not with this tree! We hardly said a word. The Christmas music was playing. The look on Pete's face of contentment and joy is still a picture in my mind, like a favorite photograph that captured a special moment.

Chemotherapy with CPT-11 through an IV continued every other week. Mary Jo came with us each time, and helped with transporting Pete. He had diarrhea attacks during the chemo treatment pretty regularly. Bill and Nan joined us, and the angels were always present in the treatment room with Pete. Bill had asked God if he should find a more experienced healer to work with Pete. Bill got the message that God would guide him and show him what to do. I had a dread that the CPT-11 wasn't working. Pete's symptoms kept getting worse.

Pete was now dependent on me for almost all the tasks of daily living. He continued with his graciousness in his dependence, though it had to be excruciating for him. His peace, appreciation and courage, I took as signs of God's presence within him and with me.

I started losing weight at a rate of about a pound a week. My boundless energy had finally found a good use. But it was hard physical work. We had some angry moments. The doctor had prescribed Questran, a powder to put in Pete's drinks to help control his diarrhea. Pete hated it. He resisted drinking it. The fights we used to have, when he resisted taking his medicine, began again. It was late one night, and he had refused the Questran all day. His diarrhea came back in full force and he had made a mess all over himself.

"This is why you take the Questran," I said angrily. "You hate the diarrhea and I hate cleaning it up."

"I'm sorry. I'm sorry," Pete said pitifully.

"I just want you to make the connection between the two things. Stop whining about taking the Questran, or you can clean up your own shit from now on," I said angrily.

Pete got admitted to the hospital emergency room the next night. His blood pressure had spiked, and his primary care doctor, Dr. Smith, was not willing to just treat the high blood pressure. They did a CAT scan and saw no bleeding or swelling. But they wanted him to spend the night. They admitted him and increased his steroids. I was surprised we ended up in the hospital. I had not expected that outcome. Pete didn't want to be there.

The doctors the next day did an MRI, and concluded that Pete might have had a minor stroke based on something they saw in the MRI. Pete was sure he didn't have a stroke. He said he got himself to the hospital by "taking a break" for the day. He hadn't slept well, and I had gotten mad at him, and that combination landed him here. I called Steve and Michael to tell them. Steve said, "This is the beginning of the end." I felt like a knife had just gone though my heart. At the same time, I knew he probably was right.

Pete stayed only twenty-four hours in the hospital. We were happy to get home. I wondered to God what was this all about. I remember crawling into Pete's arms in bed the night we got home, and after entrusting both of us in prayer to God, I felt a peace and a sense of His presence with us now in a very special and intimate way.

It turned out that Pete was right about not having a stroke. The residents who interpreted the MRI were wrong, but later Dr. Albright did confirm that though Pete didn't have a stroke that night, he had probably had a slight stroke in the occipital lobe of the brain, which affects vision. It probably happened sometime during the month of October. Dr. Albright said the Avastin might have caused it. It was now just showing up on Pete's MRI in December.

Pete and I had decided to mat and frame the Le Mans posters we had received at the race in June for Christmas presents for Michael and Steve. We put a picture of Pete with the appropriate son in the matting with each poster. Pete had gotten all of our framing work done. He used a store near his office, which did good work for a reasonable rate. Pete wanted to go with me to Bud's with the posters and pictures in hand. I was lucky and got a parking spot right in front of the shop.

Pete slowly got out of the car. He wanted to walk into Bud's shop. He didn't want to use the wheelchair. I think those few steps out of the car, slowly and laboriously across the sidewalk, and up the step to Bud's shop, were the most painful steps of Pete's whole journey. But it was worth it. It was Christmas, and this trip was for Michael and Steve's Christmas present! Bud tenderly and kindly helped Pete place the order. Bud made sure he understood Pete's desire for format and frame. Pete was very engaged. He picked out what he wanted with few words, but lots of pointing. Bud smiled and Pete smiled back a grin of utter satisfaction.

A couple of days later, Pete, in his wheelchair this time, rolled into the Good Samaritan Cancer Treatment Center with Montgomery Inn rib dinners for the cancer care staff and Dr. Albright. Pete was like he was when he was healthy, his face full of light and smiles. There he was, shaking hands and thanking them and sharing Merry Christmas wishes to all the staff. The hospital staff didn't get treated like this very often! Pete was the hero of the day!

Mary Jo came over and we went Christmas shopping, which was a wonderful break for me. Mike stayed with Pete and they watched the movie *Green Beret*. That night we went to Bella Luna's, a favorite Italian restaurant of Pete's, which we had frequented many times.

Harry, the owner, loved Pete, and showed him such affection and kindness. Pete was in his wheelchair this visit, and Harry started kidding him about flirting with the girls. He told Pete he was a dangerous driver in that chair and was a threat to his other guests. Pete was grinning from ear to ear. So was Harry. What fun we had that night!

I apologized to Pete for getting angry at him the night before he went into the hospital. I was wrong to be angry. I begged his forgiveness. "I am sorry I have been pushing you so hard on taking the Questran and doing your exercises."

My apology meant a lot to him. He didn't say much right away, but talked about it again at dinner. He wanted to know who I had talked to that gave me a change in heart. "Mean," he said. "You have been being mean to me."

I was broken by his words. I was trying to love him, and all he experienced was my meanness. He was so sincere and transparent. His words were genuine. I knew I could be mean. I asked Pete again for his forgiveness. "I am so sorry, Pete. I am so sorry." I said in tears. "I didn't intend to be mean. Can you forgive me?"

"I'm working on it," Pete said. "I am not there yet."

"Do you want to trade me in for someone new?" I asked.

His face got soft. "No. You are wonderful. I don't want to leave you. I love you more than anyone."

As I reflected on being mean, I understood that when I was afraid, I exerted pressure. Pete didn't respond well to pressure. Mary Jo had helped me see that I needed to back off. "Let Pete alone," she had told me. "Stop pushing him." I saw the truth of what she said immediately. She was once again an angel of God to me. I began repeating to myself during the day Jesus' words to his friends: "Do not let your hearts be troubled, and do not be afraid."

I realized that life was indeed tragic. It was full of suffering. I needed to embrace the suffering. My suffering; Pete's suffering. I had to stop fighting it. Pete was a victim of a cruel and ugly disease. This disease did not come from God. Disease and death were not part of God's original plan. God could redeem this suffering by His presence, just like Jesus did when faced with disease and death when he was on this earth. The redemption came in His presence with us—within Pete. I saw evidence all the time—and within me—and between us. By trusting, loving, being joyful, being hopeful, this disease did not conquer Pete. It didn't conquer me. God was glorified in the process. In our journey. And that was the only thing that mattered.

More and more of the things that Pete loved were getting beyond his reach. He couldn't read the newspaper at all anymore, not even the headlines. I poured him a glass of his favorite wine at dinner, and it would sit at his side untouched all night. He was still easily touched by others' kindness. He was so transparent. How I loved the beauty of his genuineness. Betty wrote him a thank-you note for going to her birthday party, and Pete's eyes filled with tears. Joe, his friend who also had a brain tumor, was hospitalized. The day after Pete got home from his hospital stay, we were on our way back to the hospital to visit Joe. Pete was in his wheelchair, and Joe was sitting in his hospital chair. The look of tenderness on both of their faces showed such compassion and understanding between the two. Pete prayed for Joe each morning asking God to "Give Joe more days, Lord."

TV had now become Pete's only comfort, and to make that work, Pete would close his right eye, and watch with only his left eye open. I would watch him watching the TV with his face contorted to keep that right eye closed, slumped over in his wheelchair. It was excruciating. I was losing him by inches. Each inch was painful.

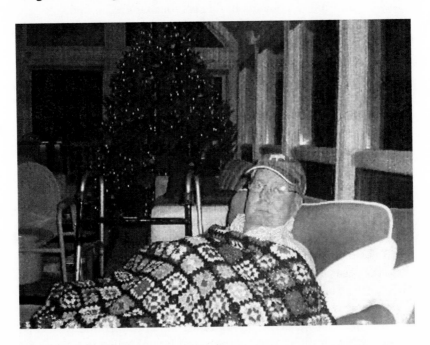

Pete and the Christmas tree—in his favorite chair

Pete's Carepage: December 12, 2007 @ 6:13 PM EST

Pete in his favorite place... overlooking the Ohio River with a warm afghan his mother made, and the Christmas tree burning bright. When the sun is out (lots of gray days in Ohio lately) it is even better!

Extreme sluggishness and additional weakness in that right side seems to be the consequence of the earlier stroke. The CT scan showed that no bleeding had occurred (thank God again) and the MRI showed the stroke location and the fact that the chemotherapy was continuing to get some improvement for Pete. Once again, not a HUGE improvement, but no new growth and the diseased area a little less dense. The doc told us that the Avastin, which Pete is getting with the chemo, could have been a contributing factor to the stroke, since it affects blood supply. Pete decided to continue to "stay the course" with the current chemo treatment, even with the risk of future strokes, since the effectiveness of the chemo moves to over fifty percent with the Avastin and drops to twenty to thirty percent without it. As Pete said, "This is no decision. Let's move ahead."

Pete is becoming weaker and weaker. He has difficult days when he can't get his foot or leg to follow his order to move. It just won't. Everything takes a lot of effort. But Pete still wants to get out. We made it to a bank Christmas party and dinners with friends, and the Christmas symphony show is planned for this weekend. He still doesn't complain, just gets a little more frustrated these days (as do I). He is one gutsy fighter, and his courage and determination continue to amaze.

I was telling friends how peaceful and full of gratitude Pete is. He is easily touched by the smallest kindness shown him, and even with the constraints he has, he appreciates every day. I love getting him up in the morning! The look on his face is so special—he is thanking God for waking up! And I am so aware of God's presence in him through these simple things. This independent entrepreneur who is used to controlling and driving everything is getting God's special blessings and he is indeed transformed. (Not that he is NOT a stubborn patient at times, too!) As he reminded me as I made plans for us to go out and celebrate the two year anniversary of his diagnosis: "It's not a two-year anniversary celebration. I am beginning my third year! That's what we will celebrate!" Ah, that's Pete!

We are looking forward to a wonderful Christmas surrounded by family. New Year's, when we go to a different city each year with our

longtime (fifteen years now) special New Year's Eve friends, will be at
our house in Cincinnati this year. Pajama party time as Judith would
say!

We wish you a Merry Christmas and Good New Year, too. You are
in our hearts as we thank God for this year—all those mornings of
waking up! You helped make those happen. Just perfectly.

Keep praying that the chemo and Avastin will kill this tumor, and
that Pete would be safe from any danger in receiving the treatments.
Pray for his strength, so that his body can withstand this onslaught,
and pray that God's purposes may be done.

A month after Mike built Pete's steps to help him get into our platform bed in our bedroom, the steps to get down to that bedroom
became too difficult for Pete. We moved upstairs again to sleep. By
mid-December, we were going down those stairs from our makeshift
bedroom to our living area, by sitting and bumping one step at a time,
his wheelchair waiting for us at the bottom of the six steps.

On December 15, 2007, Pete fell and I could not lift him. Mary Jo
and Mike came over to help me assess the situation and get Pete up.
We decided it was time to get a hospital bed in our living room, so
Pete wouldn't have to maneuver any stairs. It was snowing, and it was
a Saturday. The medical equipment supply house delivered Pete's
new bed within hours. I was impressed with the service. And thankful. God's angels. We had had tickets that night to the Cincinnati
Symphony Christmas show. They went unused. We didn't make it
outside the house again for a social event.

Dr. Smith, our primary care physician, shared with me that Dr.
Albright had just called him and shared with him Pete's MRI results,
and said the "prospects look pretty bad." I hung up from that call so
depressed. This is it, I guess. This is how it is done. Dr. Albright was
making a handoff to our primary care doctor, because he was thinking
that he couldn't do much more for Pete. He was getting Dr. Smith
ready to handle all the last details. Dr. Smith had kindness in his
voice. I thanked him for the call.

From my prayer journal: December of 2007.

Well, the medical guys are all giving up! I know you are bigger
than the medical guys. Didn't Martha say to you when Lazarus died,
"If only you had been here, my brother would not have died." Show
up now, Lord! Show up NOOOWWW!

Mary Jo, Mike and Steve all believe that Pete is starting the
"beginning of the end." All physical evidence would point to this

truth. I want to accept the truth and reality, because you are truth, not deception. It surely doesn't seem like you are going to heal Pete. It's not my job to ask you why. I also know you are not always revealed in common sense conclusions. You are bigger than medical reality. Sometimes you wait. And you ask us to wait. I accept the truth and reality as I know it.

I also still believe that you could still heal Pete. It only takes your word. Your word creates. I believe in your word and your power. He is suffering so, Lord. Deliver Pete from his enemies. They are closing in on him on every side. Come and do not delay! You could show Your glory by restoring him. You hate disease, Lord. You healed thousands when you were here. Pete has a horrible disease. He can't express himself.

I know you know his heart, Lord. And whatever your purposes are, I accept, so be it. Your kingdom come, not mine. But I'll keep asking, like you told us to. I don't know what to pray now. Come Holy Spirit, intercede for Pete because I have no words left. I don't know what to utter. Pray for Pete for me. May you be glorified in Pete and my journey. Stay with us. We need you.

23

The Last Dance

Our living space was now Pete's bedroom. The head of his hospital bed was next to the window with the view of the river. We kept his favorite chair next to the bed. Wade, our physical therapist, taught us how to make transfers easily between the bed and the chair. Pete now had no more stairs to navigate. No more worries. Peace. I slept on our couch or on the inflated air mattress my sister Beth had lent us. We rented a hospital table that made it easier for Pete to eat from his bed or chair. I'd put his portable mirror that he used to trim his moustache on that table, and he could shave himself and brush his teeth in the morning.

The Christmas tree towered over us both, beautiful with its lights and smells. Pete helped me send our Christmas cards. He was a little slow in processing how to seal and stamp the envelopes at first, but soon it came to him, and he was working right beside me. He helped with Christmas present wrapping.

Chemotherapy occurred every other Thursday. Mary Jo went with us and helped me, since Pete usually had multiple diarrhea attacks while hooked up to the IV. Bill and Nan came each time faithfully, and Michael the archangel was Pete's constant companion, a fellow warrior in the treatment room. Bill told me that Pete's aura had crept up to the top of his head, and was not protecting the rest of his body. Bill got Pete's aura re-centered. But I remembered what that meant.

Bill had told me months ago that a person's aura climbs up their body and moves beyond it completely, when they die.

Pete was miserable. The diarrhea was really bad. It was not unusual for us to have to change his clothes up to three times a day. Sometimes we also had to wash the bed linens, or the protective covering I had put on Pete's chair. The laundry was a constant task for me.

Pete was angry one morning and in his frustration, he threw away his silverware, and ate his breakfast with his fingers. Pete was fastidious in his grooming habits and his table manners. He would regularly correct me if I had violated etiquette. My heart broke again.

Michael came in for Christmas on Saturday, December 22. He got in late. His father's face lit up in delight, the only time Pete looked happy that whole day. That evening, Pete got very sick. He became incontinent twice that night, waking himself up. He had stomach pains and constant hiccups. He groaned in agony. In the morning, Pete's blood pressure registered a very low 78/59. Pete could hardly keep himself seated upright at the dining room table, because he was so weak. I felt panic. Michael came upstairs.

"Michael, I can't get a reading on his blood sugar. It just keeps reading high no matter how many times I take it," I said, pointing to the blood sugar testing instrument. "I don't want to keep sticking your dad. Can you look at this brochure and see if you can find a phone number to call to figure out what this means?" I asked with fear rising in my voice.

Michael moved into action fast. He started working the manufacturer of the blood sugar tool on the internet and the phone, while I kept calling Pete's doctor. As it always happens, it was Sunday morning and doctors are hard to find. Michael got someone on the phone from the manufacturer of the blood sugar tool.

"They said when it is registering 'high' that means your blood sugar is above 500 and the instrument can't measure any higher," Michael blurted out.

"Normal blood sugar would be about 90," I said.

My fears got worse. Pete's head fell to his chest.

Albright called back. "Let's don't risk riding this out," Dr. Albright said. "I know it is Christmas, but get him into the emergency room and I'll be by to see him tomorrow."

That was at eleven a.m. By twelve-thirty p.m. Michael, Pete and I were in the hospital. Pete's blood sugar registered 511. He was dehydrated and his heart showed afibrillation. They started an IV and a cardiac drip. Pete was hooked up to heart monitors.

Michael left the hospital to pick up Steve and Kathy, who were flying in from Washington DC for Christmas. As a family, we ended up spending all of Sunday, December 23 in the emergency room watching the Tampa Bay Buccaneers, with their dad going in and out of alertness. The hours stretched on. We gave thanks for a TV and the chance to watch Michael's team. Good distraction. Pete got into a hospital room late that night.

Christmas Eve was all about heart specialists trying to determine the cause and the treatment options for Pete's atrial fibrillation. Fibrillation meant that Pete's heartbeat was irregular, beating at a more rapid pace than normal. Was it the steroids causing the fibrillation? Was it the blood sugar? Was it Avastin? The hospitalist doctor, Dr. Dickens, told me Pete would be here for awhile. My spirit sank.

Dr. Dickens finally figured out what was wrong with Pete long after Christmas had come and gone. The diarrhea from his chemotherapy treatments had caused severe dehydration; the dehydration spiked Pete's blood sugar, and that high of a blood sugar did bad things to anybody's body. In Pete's case, it affected his heart.

Dr. Albright gave us his Christmas present when he came by to see Pete on Christmas Eve and told us that, "If Pete didn't have bad luck, he'd had no luck at all." I just looked at him in sadness. There was nothing wrong with Pete's heart. Once the blood sugar got under control, his fibrillation stopped.

We got home from the hospital Saturday, December 29, 2007. He had been in the hospital all of Christmas week. Both sons had returned to their homes by the time we got home

Christmas Day in the hospital was eerie. It was very quiet. The drive to the hospital Christmas morning felt sacred to me. I was alone. With Kathy, Steve and Michael, we had celebrated Christmas the night before in Pete's hospital room. They cooked prime rib, as Michael said, "at flashpoint," and brought it to their Dad's hospital room with all the fixings. Steve had pulled a bottle of his dad's favorite Plumpjack wine out of the wine rack, and we had a feast around Pete's hospital bed. We opened our Christmas presents for each other.

Kathy had built a bound book titled "The Nadherny Family's Visit to Le Mans." It was a beautiful and fantastic gift of photos of our trip, with funny and affectionate descriptions all bound together in a hardbound book. We were all touched and delighted by the memory of that past June. Both sons were touched by Pete's gift to them, the Le

Mans poster with their photo with him. Kathy had brought us a Josh Groban Christmas CD. The Christmas songs played. We made that hospital room festive, and no hospital staff bothered us for hours. Mary Jo and Mike stopped by to share a glass of wine. The look of sadness in Pete's eyes that Christmas Eve night still haunts me.

Pete's Carepage: December 26, 2007 at 9:47 PM EST

Quick update and a request as ever for your prayers.

Pete spent Christmas in the hospital. He is still there. He is very sick. His blood pressure spiked and his blood sugars were "off the charts." Went into the emergency room on 12/23. He is very sad. Both sons were in for Christmas and we ended up spending it in the hospital. Ugh. But we made the most of it—Mike cooked prime rib the "fast way," we had candles and Christmas music playing and wonderful gifts for each other—none surpassing the amazing love within that hospital room.

Pete is feeling that he doesn't want to fight any more. I respect his desires. Over the next few days we will make some decisions about whether to continue treatment or not. We need to "test" his feelings and make sure they are truly reflective of what he wants. It's made all the more difficult by his inability to communicate well.

So please pray that we make the right decisions about Pete's future. Pray that God's presence is with Pete and with me. Someone told me once "where there is life, there is hope." And I have hope. God has been "our path" through this whole journey. I know He is continuing to lead us and we want to follow! I continue to be bold asking God for Pete's healing and restoration. Join with me in being relentless in our asking, just like the widow! Pete and I put our trust in Him. His presence and his peace are with us.

P.S. Thanks to so many of you for your cards/gifts/flowers and good wishes for the holidays. Jesus does surprise us all the time!

§ § § § § §

My prayers go out to you
Grant Youngman, December 27, 2007 at 12:48 PM EST

Pete and Kathy,

I am so sorry and yet so uplifted by your news. You face such a difficult time, which saddens me so, and yet you have God's grace in dealing with it. Whatever you do, I am sure it will be God's will. The uplifting affirmation of faith throughout your letters and prayers, and all of the wishes and prayers of your friends and family, are a blessing to all of us. I hope you know this and it gives you some comfort in this painful phase.

God bless you both with the strength and wisdom to deal with whatever happens—a miraculous healing or a miraculous return for Pete to the heavenly Father, and the continuation of understanding, faith, and love that you have shown and received, Kathy.

Grant Youngman

Depression flooded over Pete. His sons were in. It was Christmas, and he was caught captive in this hospital room. Pete refused his medicine. I was now totally out of control. I couldn't influence Pete. He couldn't communicate. I didn't know if his refusal of medicine was his stubbornness or despair. I prayed with desperation. Perhaps refusal of his medicine was his last source of control.

"I give up," he said. "Just let me go home. I'm ready to die."

Pete was very sluggish, but all his vital signs were improving. As his blood sugar came down, his afib stopped. Heart rate normalized. We finally got home Saturday afternoon, December 29. His two cousins from Chicago drove down for a short visit that day. Bountiful food was being delivered to our home by many friends. Friends and family visited us regularly at the hospital and at home. Pete took his medicine without a fight the day before we got home. Things were improving.

Pete's Carepage: January 03, 2008 @ 7:41 PM EST

Thanks to all of you who "stormed the heavens" for Pete and me over the Christmas holidays. You got us home! We made it out of the hospital the evening of December 29 and Pete was "happy, happy." He just kept saying that one word as he sat in his wheelchair and took in the view of the Ohio River from our living room. Once Pete's blood sugars got under control, his heart went back to normal rhythm and after a couple of units of blood to "pump" him up, we got cut loose!

Our friends still came into Cincinnati for our sixteenth annual New Year's get-together and the posted picture is New Year's Day in our kitchen, cooking dinner. Judith cooked all of Pete's favorite things: homemade crab soup and salmon on the grill. A fire burned in our fireplace all weekend, and snow fell lightly outside. Our best wines from our cooler were drunk all day and night. Friend Mike M. pulled

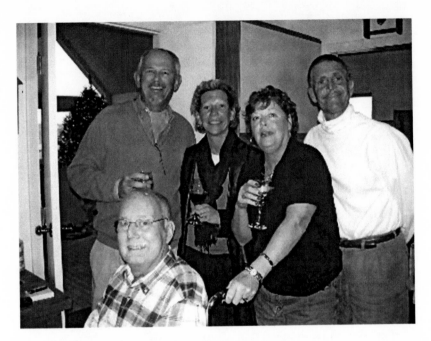

Jack, Pam, Mike, and Judith on Pete's last New Year's Eve

*out all of Pete's favorite CDs. Mike on the floor and Pete next to him
in his wheelchair moving in rhythm for hours to Steely Dan and the
Rolling Stones and Creedence and the Doobie Brothers. Pete was so
happy. All of a sudden it was midnight. Pete was going strong. We
kissed in 2008! Happy New Year! Friends loving each other. On the
journey together. Joy was in our house that weekend.*

*Today we got the results of a new MRI. Pete's neuro-oncologist
said Pete is holding his own. The doctor described the situation as a
"stalemate," meaning that the tumor is not growing but it is also not
shrinking. He advised, and Pete is in agreement, to continue the
chemo treatments but at a reduced level. Hopefully, the tumor can
stay contained with less chemo and Pete will suffer less damaging
side effects. The doctor confirmed that Pete's body is very fragile and
can't take any more aggressive action now. Pete's spirits are doing
better since he got home. He hates that hospital. His humor is returning and he is smiling more, even though still very weak and
exhausted. When he prays, he can only get out a few words—but I
hear him once again say "thanks" in appreciation of the day.*

*So our request of you is to pray for Pete's body to regain strength
so he can withstand the next chemo treatment, which is scheduled for*

January 10. It clearly looks like any healing that the medicine can provide is less and less. God sometimes answers us when human actions are impossible. So be bold with us and ask God for his healing hand to be on Pete. Ask Him to battle this tumor in Pete and bring him to recovery. Jesus has been our path during this journey. We are following Him and we ask that He be glorified in our circumstance!

After the holidays, my friends at the United Way's Women Leadership Council started bringing us food two or three times a week. That was a huge relief for me, and a comfort. On one such occasion, Pete had fallen. I had called my brother Brian to come over to help us get back in the chair. While we waited for him, I sat down on the floor next to Pete. His mother's afghan covered his shoulders and kept him from getting a chill. We just sat on the floor right next to each other. Our United Way friend Cynthia knocked on the door with our dinner for the night. I called for her to come in. There Pete and I were, on the floor, smiling. I explained our situation. She sat for a moment. We laughed together. And I thought how exposed we were. There was no private place. No hiding. We would have been embarrassed years before to be found in such a predicament. Now it was just fine.

Pete's eyes were full of appreciation as he looked at me as I sat with him on the floor. He was not alone. Our strong bond was evident. Kindness and love between us. And peacefulness. That was how our days had been since he got home from the hospital. I felt no fear. We were totally focused on each other. I felt so honored to be in such a position to be with Pete in this way. How privileged I truly was.

A couple of things converged that January of 2008. Our Crossroads friend, Jerry, came over and prayed with us. He was on the spiritual Board of Governors of Crossroads, and his visit meant a lot to both of us.

He asked for "peace and blessing in our home created by God's presence." He asked God to "provide His healing touch to every cell within Pete's body." I was glad for Jerry's prayer, and Betty's homemade soup that he brought with him.

Then a friend of Pete's, who was a brain tumor survivor of five years, sent him this note.

January 03, 2008

Dear Kathy,

Pete has been on my mind ever since your last Carepage. I do not have words to express my feelings

*the way I should, but Pete has been an inspiration
to me through his courage and internal strength. At
my church, he has been put in the "book of inten-
tions" that are prayed for at every mass. It is a
little thing, but the members understand the power
of prayer.*

*Tell Pete that I am looking forward to the fishing
trip that we are going to have next spring on the
Ohio River.*

*Finally, Jim Valvano, a famous basketball coach
who died in 1993 from cancer, said "I know, I gotta
go, I gotta go, and I got one last thing and I said
it before, and I want to say it again. Cancer can
take away all of my physical abilities. It cannot
touch my mind, it cannot touch my heart and it cannot touch my soul. And those three things are going
to carry on forever.*

I thank you and God bless you all."

Please keep in touch.

Jim

Pete cried as I read him Jim's message.

Finally, an old friend of mine from high school, Tom, who now lived in New Hampshire, sent us a book called *Learning to Fall* by Phil Simmons. Through contact with my family, Tom knew of Pete's illness and had followed us on Pete's Carepage. Phil Simmons, a friend of Tom's, had a terminal illness, ALS (amyotropic lateral scle-rosis, known as Lou Gehrig's disease). I read and loved the book. I told Pete that chapter two, "Getting Up in the Morning," reminded me of him. He said to read it to him. He closed his eyes and listened to the whole chapter. That was rare, given his short attention span. He really liked it.

A section of that chapter is as follows:

"My diagnosis doesn't make me special. Life, as I have said
before, is a terminal condition. Those of us with terminal diseases
simply have been blessed—and I mean blessed—with having the
facts of our own mortality held constantly before us. Death in other
words is good for us. To accept death is to live with a profound sense
of freedom. The freedom first from attachment to things of this life
that don't really matter: fame, material possessions, and even finally,
our own bodies. Acceptance brings the freedom to live fully in the
present. Only when we accept our present condition can we set aside

fear and discover the love and compassion that are our highest human endowments. And out of our compassion we deal justly with those about us. Not just on our good days, not just when it's convenient, but EVERYWHERE AND AT ALL TIMES we are free to act according to that which is highest in us. And in such action we find peace. So each day that I can get out of bed in the morning, I am blessed. Each day that any of us can move our limbs to do the world's work, we are blessed. And if limbs wither, and speech fails, we are still blessed. So long as this heart beats, I am blessed. For it is our human work, it is our human duty, finally to rise each day in the face of loss, to rise in the face of grief, of debility, of pain, to move as the turtle moves her empty nest behind her, her labor come to nothing, up out of the pit and toward the next season's doing."

Pete exemplified this principle to me. In his illness, he had taught me how to really live.

And so everything changed again for us. I crawled into the hospital bed, and into Pete's arms, and I thought about Toni's vegetable soup she had made just for us because Pete loved it so. And I thought of my niece Shauna's beef stew, and our neighbor Cheryl who brought us groceries, and Nora's Serbian soup she made from her mother's recipe, and Cynthia's manicotti and Jenny's cookies and Mary Jo and Mike's shoveling the snow and fixing the lamp that was broken in the living room. And I thought of the peace that lived between Pete and I even in this ugly situation. And I thought we are blessed! I remembered the kindness in Pete's eyes as he looked at me, and his words of appreciation. And I thought, yes Lord, your presence was here. It was enough. All that was important, more important than the question of life or death, was that we wanted you glorified in our lives. That was our mission now. Our only mission.

As we prayed one morning, Pete said, with anger in his voice, "He's coming for me and I don't want to go!" He said he had dreamed it.

"Let's pray for more days, Pete," I said. And we did.

Another morning, Pete woke up and with a great intensity told me, "It can't be a very big place! It couldn't be very big."

I wasn't sure what he saw, but he clearly saw something, given his sense of urgency. I had a sense he was describing something sacred. I stayed silent in reverence.

Jerry, Pete's best friend from Florida, came in for a short visit in the middle of January. He was not upset at all by Pete's condition. He was very comfortable in caring for Pete with me. I was thankful for him. He quieted me. Jerry had been a caregiver for his Mom and Dad, so he was comfortable with the needs Pete had. His visit was so easy. The bond of kindness and love between he and Pete was evident, as Jerry took Pete back in time, and told stories they remembered from the thirty years they had known each other. Jerry brought us fresh Florida oranges for our daily morning juice. All three of us prayed together at each meal. That was the first time we had ever prayed with Jerry.

Jerry's wife had just left him. He was full of sadness. But as he said, "It is what it is. Facts are friendly. Once I know the facts then I can deal with anything."

Jerry had learned how to fall. And he reminded Pete and me of those simple truths: "Facts are friendly. It is what it is."

Both Pete's occupational and physical therapists came to treat Pete twice a week. Every sign of strength Pete showed in his arms or leg, I would take as a sign of hope. Wade would get him walking, even if just a few steps. Chemotherapy got back on schedule, receiving a treatment on Thursday, January 17. But by the next day, Pete and I were back in the emergency room. At about three-thirty a.m., Pete was in distress. He complained once again of abdominal pain. I could not give Pete relief. His abdominal pain came in spasms. His breathing was very fast and shallow.

Pete's Carepage: January 21, 2008 @ 7:56 PM EST

This is Mary Jo & Mike on Monday evening. Kathy asked us to update Pete's Carepage. Unfortunately, Pete returned to the hospital last Friday, and Kathy has been spending most of her days (and nights) there. It's been another roller coaster ride.

Pete went in with severe pain in his abdomen, high blood pressure, rapid heartbeat, and difficulty with breathing. We found that he had fluid in his lungs, which required oxygen. However, this has been largely resolved, and he is now off of oxygen. He also had a urinary tract infection that has been resolved, and a low level of hemoglobin that has been resolved with an infusion of blood. A CAT scan also showed that Pete did not have a blockage, abscess or bleeding in his bowel—good news! However, he is still having some problems with rapid heartbeat, and the diarrhea monster has returned. He is a fighter and is working hard to get enough resolved so that he can return home.

Please pray for Pete's strength to withstand these multiple attacks on his body. Both he and Kathy are amazing in their spirit, resolve and attitude. However, they can surely use our prayers and spiritual transfusions of energy.

The scans of Pete's abdomen were normal. He didn't have a clot in his lungs, nor was pneumonia present. He had fluid in his lungs which could have been caused by the chemotherapy, the cancer, or the steroids. He had a bad first night in the hospital. When I arrived in the early morning, he was restrained and on a catheter. I got him off the catheter, and told the staff I would take charge of getting him to and from the portable toilet. I decided I wasn't leaving Pete at night anymore. I'd spend the night with him. My presence quieted him, and protected him when necessary from the nursing or lab staff's bad decisions. Paula and Mary Jo would give me relief in the morning. I'd go home and shower and pray, and then return for the rest of the day.

From my prayer journal: January 19–20, 2008

O Father. We come to you. Help. We are in your hands. You are our path. You have Pete and me in your hands. You have stripped all things away. We rely on you.

Your child, Pete, is very sick. He is in the hospital. Thank You for protecting him from a clot and pneumonia. He has fluid in his lungs and is on oxygen. Help him, Lord. Send your presence to him. Your healing touch. It sure seems like you are not going to intervene in healing Pete. I accept your silence. I accept your purposes. But I keep asking, Lord. You told us to be bold. Ask in your name. You are our path. We follow you on this journey. Pete declines more and more. The cancer and the chemo wrack his body. He is suffering so. Do not abandon us. Deliver Pete from his enemies. We have not earned your grace or mercy. We are not worthy. But your mercy you have given. Have mercy on us.

There is not a lot more that the doctors can do. They are working hard to solve this last puzzle, but I hear resignation in their voices. Resignation rings in Mary Jo and Paula's voices, too. Pete is dying. Perhaps the fight is up. Death lurks at his edges. You, Lord, are the source of life. We hang on your balance. You are El-Shaddai. The Lord Almighty. You create and you take away. We accept your purposes. Pete is in your hands, Lord. Take good care of him. Wrap your arms around him and let him know the wonderful comfort of your presence and love. May your glory be shown in our circumstance.

Pete's hospital room was filled with visitors. Kevin and Ann Marie, Dolan, Dianne, Missy, Cathy, Nan and Bill, Tony and Karen, Paula and Robin. How blessed Pete and I were!

Missy told me, "Keep asking, Kath, keep asking. Don't give up!"

Dianne had been recruited by Pete at Makro over twenty-five years ago. Dianne and I had been good friends. She lived with me for a while as she went through her own transition years ago. She had been one of the few friends invited to our wedding. We had lost touch. Now she reappeared, hearing of Pete's illness from one of Pete's customers. Pete had a huge grin for her as she walked into his hospital room. He could not speak. But he winked at her. Later, she told me, she got that wink and with it a silent but clear request from Pete to "take care of me." And she has.

Pete's Carepage: January 24, 2008 @ 8:23 AM EST

Pete made it home from the hospital last night. Faster than we had expected, although too slow for Pete. He got his "feistiness" back yesterday and began asking every hospital staff person he saw when he could get home! After another setback on Tuesday when we found two blood clots in Pete's right thigh and calf, the doctors decided that he was protected enough by a blood clot filter that had been inserted back in the spring of 2006. After some blood thinner and a new "sock" to help his circulation, he was good to go! The Lord is good. Thank you for lifting us again in your prayers and not giving up on us. So many more serious obstacles the docs were worried about, like pneumonia or a clot in Pete's lung, were again diverted. Talk about deliverance!

So we are home. Todd, a friend from Minneapolis and US Banker, was in town and planning a visit last night, so along with my sister and brother-in-law, Mary Jo and Mike (ever-faithful angels!) we got Pete home and witnessed that smile of his when he got wheeled into his home. Pure joy!

Continue to pray for Pete's strength to recover. He is very weak. He will skip the next chemo treatment that was scheduled for today, and let his body renew itself. Pray for Pete and for all involved in his care that we listen and get God's guidance as to when to resume treatment. And we thank you for your belief and your intercession on our behalf. We continue to rely on your prayers for us while on this journey.

The very evening that we got home from the hospital, Pete's pain returned while he was sleeping. He was afraid. I crawled into his bed with him. My body seemed to calm him.

"What is wrong? What is the cause of this pain?" Pete asked me.

I reassured him that the scans had not shown anything wrong with his abdomen. Other than that, I had no good answers. I was afraid. I remembered the Lord's words and repeated them over and over: "Do not let your heart be troubled or afraid. Trust in me. I am here." I gave Pete some Tylenol and a heating blanket and he quieted. He brushed my cheek with his hand and thanked me for everything.

The next morning, Mary Jo and Mike came over to keep vigil. Such comfort to both of us! Nora brought us some groceries. I ran out to the pharmacy to get Pete's prescriptions. A friend from the Women's Leadership Council dropped dinner off. Mary Jo, Mike and I sat near Pete's bed and fed him chicken, asparagus, mashed potatoes and milk. He ate well. And he slept well the night of January 25. Mary Jo spent the night with us. I slept well next to Pete.

Mike was back at the house by eight a.m. on January 26, and shortly after Mike returned, Pete started moaning again. His pain was intense. He sipped some milk. It seemed the only thing that comforted him. He was breathing from his abdomen with rapid respirations of about forty-six a minute. Mary Jo was counting. Pete's blood pressure had spiked to 180/110. I called Dr. Smith's office. No response. A half hour passed. I called again. The doctor covering for Dr. Smith called back and said to get Pete to the emergency room. My heart was broken again. I talked to Pete.

"The doctor wants you back into the emergency room. I am so sorry, honey. I don't know what else to do. Mary Jo and I can't figure out how to give you any relief from this pain. I know you don't want to go. But we don't know what else to do. I think we should go back to the hospital."

Pete nodded his head in agreement. The ambulance arrived. I rode in the back with him next to the stretcher.

We went through the same routine in the emergency room we had gone through before. Pete got strong pain medicine that knocked him out. Dr. Dickens came in, and gave him another drug to get him alert. It worked. The scans showed no abdominal obstruction.

Mary Jo and Mike had a dinner date that Saturday night. I told them to go ahead and go. My brother Brian came to be with me. He brought some dinner. We went to get a CT scan of Pete's lungs just to make sure a clot had not moved near his heart or lungs. The dye injected into Pete's vein for the scan blew up in Pete's arm. The dye never made it to his heart or lungs, so the scan couldn't be taken. I asked if they could try again. They couldn't do another scan since Pete had had three doses of dye in twenty-four hours, and any more dye would have been dangerous. They would need to wait until tomorrow. We waited patiently for a room.

At about seven-thirty p.m., Pete started getting worse. His respirations increased to between fifty-six and seventy-one a minute. His blood pressure was back up to 140/84 and his oxygen level dropped to eighty-one even though he was on oxygen. The nurse in the emergency room changed Pete's room request from a regular floor to an intensive care room. Brian called Mary Jo and Mike and told them to come back to the hospital. They called Nan and Bill. Paula was working, but I was in phone contact with her about every fifteen minutes. My sister Beth arrived.

I called both boys. I got hold of Steve, who was battling a cold and therefore home on a Saturday night. I left a message for Michael with the news that his dad had gotten worse, and to call me as soon as possible. While talking to Steve, I put the phone up to Pete's ear so Pete could hear Steve's voice. I could see the trace of recognition and love for Steve in Pete's eyes.

About eight-thirty p.m. Pete turned his face to mine. Our eyes locked. Everything in that emergency room—all the noise and chaos of an urban hospital on a Saturday night—faded from my view and ears. Calm descended. For the next two hours we didn't move our gaze from each other.

I told him how I loved him. I told him how God loved him even more than me. I told him to rest. I prayed with him, and asked the Holy Spirit to pray the words for me for Pete. I realized now that Pete was dying.

I had his right hand in mine. My left hand caressed his neck and face. I kept smiling and winking at Pete, just like we always did when we were having a great time together. I knew Pete was dying, and I noticed how strange it was that I kept smiling. I couldn't stop smiling; it wasn't forced. It was a genuine, loving, happy smile like I would get when I'd see him after being away for a few days. The smile kept coming to my face again and again. I thought, *Where is this smile coming from?*

And then I knew! Pete loved my smile. He loved to have me smile at him. It was the very favorite thing he loved about me. He'd try to make me smile when I was mad or sad. And he knew he was leaving. He wanted a last snapshot. Me smiling was the last picture he wanted. A single tear rolled down from his cheek. I knew he was sad to leave me. We never said good-bye.

And then he was gone. I saw or maybe I heard him go. It was both—seeing and hearing, but not exactly either. A powerful, strong force like a wind. It went out from him through the right side of his face. I knew he was gone. The doctors came in and confirmed his death.

Epilogue

This is the last update to our Carepage. As many of you know, Pete died at 10:35 on Saturday night, January 26, in the emergency room of Good Samaritan hospital. It all seemed very fast to me. But Pete and I were blessed in this last step of his journey, just as we have been blessed throughout.

I was trying to think of what Pete would want to say to all of you. You the faithful followers of ours—throughout these last two years— OR as Pete corrected me, "I am beginning my third year!" He would say thank you. Over and over and over again. Thanks for the love. Thanks for the belief in him and me. Thanks for all the support. Thanks for all the messages. Thanks for all the cards. As I would read him your messages, he would get "teary," so touched by your kindness and your love of him. And he would get frustrated because he couldn't write or talk back to you. So I suspect Pete IS talking NOW! You may get some pent-up messages from him! And some delayed reaction from those of you with such bad jokes/humor.

I am so happy and thankful that God allowed us to share all the last moments together. He went into the emergency room on Saturday morning with the same abdominal pain that had disappeared during the last hospital stay. We kept him at home as long as we could until Tylenol and Percocet couldn't give him any more relief. So in the emergency room they got Pete some pain medicine by noon. He seemed to be recovering. The scans of his chest and abdomen showed no problems. The doc was going to admit him and continue to search

263

for the source of the pain. Then, Pete started to have very labored breathing and a very fast and high heart rate. The doc had decided that he didn't need another scan of his lungs even though he had blood clots in his legs; he had a filter that would protect him from those clots moving to his lungs/heart. But the filter wasn't 100% and he seemed to have the symptoms of just that. Another scan was attempted but it failed. It began to be apparent that Pete was fighting hard but couldn't get stable. He looked at me and his eyes would stay fixed on me for the next couple of hours. Son Steve was able to call and talk to his dad, and I could tell from Pete's eyes that Pete could hear him and was comforted. All the noise and chaos of an emergency room on a Saturday night in an urban hospital faded from my view. I stopped looking at the monitor and I met Pete's gaze and for the next couple of hours we danced our last dance together. I told him all the things I wanted to say about how loved he was; how he had saved my life a few times and how thankful I was for him; Pete was surrounded by family and our healer Bill and his wife Nan—and I could whisper to him that I knew God loved him more than all these people combined! And he could rest now, and not fight or work so hard. I never saw fear in his eyes. Just peace and calm. And then he was gone. We never said good-bye. We will see each other again.

I chose the readings for the celebration service we will have for Pete this week. Our neighbor led me to the right passage. Our neighbor said, "I could hear God in a booming voice welcoming Pete with the words of Matthew 25:23: 'Well done good and faithful servant. Come and share your master's happiness!'"

I was disappointed in God for not healing Pete as so many of us had prayed for. I also realize that God did heal Pete and he did restore him, just not in the way that I had hoped. And I accept and rejoice in the gift Pete was to so many of us. And we sing "Blessed be your Name" with a loud voice full of thanksgiving. Pete was always grateful for every morning that he had. How he taught us all.

PS Pete is very feisty. He has had difficulty speaking for a long time. So be alert! He just may have a few things to say to you now that he can talk again! And make sure that you laugh long and hard with him.

The night of Pete's death a couple of strange things happened. As soon as Pete died, the nursing staff, which was in tears, wheeled Pete's body into a more private place. The chaplain came down to pray with our family and friends gathered in this room. The staff kept asking me if I wanted a few minutes in private with Pete. I looked at them like they were crazy. Pete's not here! And what was so strange to me was the absolute detachment I had from Pete's body. This body, which I had been so intimate with and cared for and worried over for so long, now had no attachment for me at all. I knew Pete was gone. I had seen/heard him go. His body was just an empty shell, and I had no feeling for it whatsoever. And all the time I was feeling this, I thought it was rather weird. I kept thinking I should feel differently.

I drove myself home from the hospital. Mike and Mary Jo followed me home, and came in. Their children shortly followed and we sat on Pete's hospital bed in our living room, drinking wine.

Mike told us this story. Mike was a former math teacher and information technology senior manager for a Fortune 500 company. Which means to say, he is an analytical type and not prone to emotion or exaggeration. He felt sheepish and a little embarrassed as he spoke.

"I had a weird thing happen right after Pete's death."

We all looked at him. He had our attention. Mike had been across from me, right next to Pete—me on Pete's right side and Mike on Pete's left side for the last hours of Pete's life. Mike had Pete's left hand in his.

"I had to go the bathroom bad for the last few hours, but I wouldn't leave Pete's side. I had cased out where the closest bathroom was as I stayed near Pete. As soon as Pete died, I made a mad rush to that bathroom. I am standing at the urinal getting relief, and Pete joined me. I knew it was him. He was luminous and bright, like a brilliant light. He stood right next to me. It was him. I didn't doubt it for a minute. And he asked me if I would make sure and take care of Kathy. And of course, I said yes—and then he was gone."

There was a sense of amazement in the room. My eyes filled with tears. Pete—still worried about taking care of me! And no one else but Mike would he have entrusted to do so. They had become brothers.

I slept that night and got up early the next morning, which was my routine, to see the sunrise and pray. As I was praying, I remembered Pete's cards! Those cards he had written more than two years ago sitting in the hotel room before his first brain tumor surgery in Cleveland. He had written messages to me, Michael, Steven, his business partner Dave, and Mary Jo and Mike. He had asked me to distribute them if he didn't make it out of surgery alive. I wondered where he had put those cards. I hadn't seen them in two years. I was led to his desk. And found them easily. Covered with dust in their plastic container. I opened the box.

Pete had written a card with directions to all of us. (Only Pete!)

To All—

The cards were handy. Not a first choice but available.

And guess what.

A water view. I guess the color is appropriate (black and white photographs) but sunny and blue sky would have been my 1ˢᵗ choice.

Pete

The cards were in shiny silver envelopes. Written on the outside of mine was "Kathy."

I sat in silence, tears streaming down my face. Then, I talked right back to him. "Pete, thanks for writing all these notes. I've read mine now. I'll treasure it forever. I know all the others will be thrilled to get their note from you, too. What a kind and thoughtful thing to do. And yes, Pete—we will see each other again. And what a great day that will be!"

From my prayer journal: January 29, 2008

I give thanks to you, Lord, for Pete. What a wonderful way to show your amazing love for me. Giving me Pete! And loving Pete and honoring you all came together into one and the same dance for me—and for Pete. Amen.

Notes

Chapter 2: This Changes Everything

Living With a Brain Tumor, Peter Black (New York: Henry Holt & Company, 2006) 2:8

Brain Tumors: Finding the Ark, Paul M. Zeltzer, M.D. (California: Shilysca Press, 2006)

Brain Tumors: Leaving the Garden of Eden, Paul M. Zeltzer, M.D (California: Shilysca Press, 2004)

American Heritage Dictionary (Massachusetts: Houghton Mifflin Company, 1976) 19

Chapter 3: Diagnosis

Brain Tumors: Leaving the Garden of Eden, Paul M. Zeltzer, M.D. (California: Shilysca Press, 2004) 6:140

"FDA approves Drug for Treatment of Aggressive Brain Cancer." US Food and Drug Administration press release, May 8, 2009

Chapter 4: Second Opinion

Brain Tumors: Finding the Ark, Paul M. Zeltzer, M.D. (California: Shilysca Press, 2006) 17:27

Brain Tumors: Leaving the Garden of Eden, Paul M. Zeltzer, M.D. (California: Shilysca Press, 2004) 6:135

Chapter 5: Facing Death

Epic, John Eldredge (Tennessee: Thomas Nelson, Inc., 2004) Act Three: 72, Act Four: 73, 78–79, 87–89

Matthew 4:24
Matthew 9:2–7
Luke 7:2–9

Chapter 6: Enlisting an Army of Supporters

Jeremiah 29:11
Luke 18:1–7

Chapter 7: Surgery 1: Brain Tumor Removal

Brain Tumors: Finding the Ark, Paul M. Zeltzer, M.D. (California: Shilysca Press, 2006) 17:26

Chapter 8: Surgery 2: Clinical Trial

Brain Tumors: Leaving the Garden of Eden, Paul M. Zeltzer, M.D. (California: Shilysca Press, 2004) 3:60

Brain Tumors: Finding the Ark, Paul M. Zeltzer, M.D. (California: Shilysca Press, 2006) 21:170

Ibid, 21:170

"A Six Foot Lab Rat," Anne Underwood, Newsweek, December11, 2006

Chapter 9: The Darkest Days

Mere Christianity, C.S. Lewis (San Francisco: Harper Collins publishers, 2001 edition) 5:31

Chapter 10: Though I Walk Through the Valley of Death

Traveling Light, Max Lucado (Tennessee: W Publishing Group, Thomas Nelson, Inc., 2001) 7:59

Chapter 12: Medications and Healing Touch

Brain Tumors: Leaving the Garden of Eden, Paul M. Zeltzer, M.D. (California: Shilysca Press, 2004) 9:222

Ibid, 9:213–215

"Insurance Coverage, Medical Conditions, and Visits to Alternative Medical Providers: Results of a National Survey," Wolsko, Eisenberg, Davis, Arch Intern Medicine, 2002)

Brain Tumors: Finding the Ark, Paul M. Zeltzer M.D. (California: Shilysca Press, 2006) 18:54

"Why Does Healing Touch Work?" Colorado Center for Healing Touch Newsletter, Donald Stouffer, PhD, March 1999

Chapter 15: Living Life to the Fullest

"The Kingdom of God: Love and Judgment" Crossroads Message Outline, Greg Boyd, February 2007

Chapter 18: Living with Uncertainty

Inside Out, Larry Crabb (Colorado: Nav Press, 1988) 8:146

Chapter 20: The Last Trip

"FDA Approves Drug for Treatment of Aggressive Brain Cancer." US Food and Drug Administration press release, May 8, 2009.

Chapter 21: Doing the Dance

Mark 10:47
John 14:27

Chapter 22: The Tumor is Back

John 14:27
John 11:21
Chapter 23: The Last Dance
Learning to Fall, Philip Simmons (New York: Bantam Dell Random House, Inc, 2000) 2:20, 21, 23

All the scripture verses are from the New International Version of the Bible, International Bible Society, 1984.

CPSIA information can be obtained at www.ICGtesting.com
Printed in the USA
BVOW020710221111

276603BV00001B/31/P